Finding Meaning in the Experience of Dementia

by the same author

Palliative Care, Ageing and Spirituality
A Guide for Older People, Carers and Families
Elizabeth MacKinlay
ISBN 978 1 84905 290 0
eISBN 978 0 85700 598 4

Ageing and Spirituality across Faiths and Cultures
Edited by Elizabeth MacKinlay
ISBN 978 1 84905 006 7
eISBN 978 0 85700 374 4

Ageing, Disability and Spirituality
Addressing the Challenge of Disability in Later Life
Edited by Elizabeth MacKinlay
ISBN 978 1 84310 584 8
eISBN 978 1 84642 767 1

Spiritual Growth and Care in the Fourth Age of Life
Elizabeth MacKinlay
ISBN 978 1 84310 231 1
eISBN 978 1 84642 480 9

The Spiritual Dimension of Ageing
Elizabeth MacKinlay
ISBN 978 1 84310 008 9
eISBN 978 1 84642 037 5

Finding Meaning in the Experience of DEMENTIA

The Place of **Spiritual Reminiscence** Work

ELIZABETH MACKINLAY AND
CORINNE TREVITT

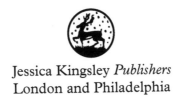

Jessica Kingsley *Publishers*
London and Philadelphia

First published in 2012
by Jessica Kingsley Publishers
116 Pentonville Road
London N1 9JB, UK
and
400 Market Street, Suite 400
Philadelphia, PA 19106, USA

www.jkp.com

Library of Congress Cataloging in Publication Data
A CIP catalog record for this book is available from the Library of Congress

British Library Cataloguing in Publication Data
A CIP catalogue record for this book is available from the British Library

ISBN 978 1 84905 248 1
eISBN 978 0 85700 657 8

Printed and bound in Great Britain

Contents

List of Figures

List of Tables

Acknowledgements

Elizabeth and Corinne would like to acknowledge and thank the following organisations and people who made this study and book possible:

The aged care organisations that provided staff, resources, access to residents and funding under the Australian Research Council (ARC) Linkage Grant (funding under Linkage Grants is provided both by the ARC and the aged care industry partners):

Anglican Retirement Community Services, Canberra and Goulburn.

Wesley Gardens UnitingCare Ageing, Sydney.

Mirinjani UnitingCare Ageing, Canberra.[1]

University of Canberra for a Collaborative Research Grant – 2001.

The ARC for a Linkage Grant – 2002–2005 (Number: LP0214980).

Professor Michael Kiernan and Karin Peters for data and statistical advice.

Our tireless research assistants and transcribers who spent hours listening to the transcripts of the spiritual reminiscence groups.

Pastoral care staff, lifestyle coordinators and diversional therapists who facilitated each of the spiritual reminiscence groups.

The participants, without whom this project would not have been possible. These people, all with diagnoses of dementia, gave generously to share their stories, both individually and in the small group settings throughout the study.

The great support of Jessica Kingsley staff in the production of this book.

Kevin Teo for his computer advice and preparation of the draft editions of this book.

---

1   The different names used at various places in the text relate to individual facilities within the organisations and also to name changes over the time since we conducted the research.

Preface

We have been privileged to travel this journey with these people who have dementia. Until the 1990s, when the late Malcolm Goldsmith wrote his ground-breaking book *Hearing the Voice of the People with Dementia* (1996), it was rare to read of or to see people with dementia being engaged in research into their condition and experience. So much has been spent on the elusive search for a cure for dementia, and yet people who have dementia need the best resources that we can provide, to be empowered to live their lives to the full, right now.

This book is the culmination of more than a decade of our research involving people with dementia. This was preceded by the beginning journey of Christine Bryden (Boden) with Elizabeth MacKinlay, as Christine was newly diagnosed with early-onset dementia. Following completion of our research, we began disseminating our work by writing a guide for care providers on our method of facilitating spiritual reminiscence with people who have dementia, subsequently translated and adapted for use in Japan.

Many of the participants, with few remaining communication skills, seemed to come alive in the interviews and small group sessions. For too long in Western societies, it seems, we have focused on what people with dementia have lost. It is time to shift the focus to look at what they still have. In the process we may find the journey less frightening and more rewarding.

We decided that Mini Mental State Examination (MMSE) scores would be mentioned in the text where these are very low or high.[1] All known scores

---

1 The Mini Mental State Examination is a short test comprising questions relating to memory, arithmetic and orientation. The MMSE is a commonly used scale for assessing cognitive status in people who may have dementia. It has a range of 0–30, and anyone with a score of 24 or below is generally deemed to have dementia. However, it is noted that, in some instances, people diagnosed with dementia may score up to 30. A MMSE score is indicative but not prescriptive of a level of cognitive impairment. As a rule the following guideline is used: patients with dementia are likely to score at least 21 on the MMSE for mild disease, 10–20 for moderate disease and 9 or less for severe disease. The MMSE score may be normal for people with early cognitive impairment (Royal Australian College of General Practitioners 2006).

of participants are listed in Appendix 2 should you wish to check the MMSE levels of particular participants.

Although some authorities have suggested that group work is not suitable for people with scores less than 24, most of the participants in our work had scores lower than this.

The material from interviews and small group sessions has been generously shared by study participants. We have assured them of their privacy and have changed all names and removed any identifying material in respect to their identities. Data drawn from the transcripts of both in-depth interviews (the one-on-one interviews) and the small group sessions is used in many places within the book. We have identified the quoted transcript by way of using 'interviewer' when it comes from an individual interview and 'facilitator' when it comes from a small group session.

The book is structured into three parts: Part 1 is Building the Evidence for Spiritual Reminiscence: Research and Theory; Part 2 is titled Listening to Those with Dementia: The Findings; and Part 3 focuses on Practice of Spiritual Reminiscence. The reader may choose where to dip into the text; however, most readers will probably find it more helpful to begin with Part 1 and Part 2 before the final part, of practice.

In Part 1 we have set out the background to the development of spiritual reminiscence and the importance of narrative or life story that underlies this. This is more than reminiscence; it is looking deeply at one's life journey, linking life-meaning with things remembered. For the person with dementia, memory itself may be a problem, and the focus of spiritual reminiscence is not simply on remembering things, but the meaning. It is important to include a chapter on current understandings of dementia. There are two definite models to consider: the biomedical model, which sees dementia as a condition to be treated and managed, while the other model is the psychosocial and spiritual model where the focus is on the person. This chapter is an important one in providing a wide lens through which to see dementia.

Part 2 begins with an examination of the person and autonomy with its relation to dementia. Ethical issues become very important in dementia because of the raised actual and potential vulnerability of the person with dementia and their family. Ethical issues arise around the topic of research too: should we do research with people who have dementia? Our answer is a clear 'Yes' and we explain why we believe this to be so.

Applying a model of the spiritual tasks and process of ageing, based on the findings from the study, we focus on seven further topics in this part of the book: issues of resilience and transcendence; humour; wisdom and insight;

dementia and multicultural issues; hope and despair; dying and death; then a final chapter in this section is a theology of dementia.

Part 3 shifts the focus again, to bring the findings to a level of practice: this is what we found – so what? Communication is obviously a vital chapter in this part. Often it is not that these people do not understand, but that it is hard for them to communicate with others; words are lost, others don't give them enough time to respond or it is so much easier to 'do for' or 'speak for' rather than give the time needed for understanding. Relationship, or connectedness with others, is almost synonymous with meaning for people with dementia. We have many examples of this in action. Another chapter on connecting through rituals, symbols and liturgy is a vital component of the book. Another chapter addresses how to design a programme for spiritual reminiscence. And a final chapter brings it all together, with issues of changing attitudes and empowering people with dementia.

We have held many workshops on spiritual reminiscence and it is being used more widely, in different countries. Over time, we have become convinced that it is important to provide a book that shares what we learnt in the process of working and researching with people who have dementia for more than eight years. We hope that our writing will shine a light into this area, which can be daunting, but also so rewarding. We are not alone in our work of seeing the person with dementia 'whole', and we could name numbers of people making valuable contributions in this field, such as Kitwood, Goldsmith, Wood, Killick, Jewell, Sabat and so many others now, who are actively working and practising in this important area.

We are extremely grateful to all those who took part in this research; their participation has enabled us to find new ways of supporting and engaging with people who have dementia in the finding of meaning in this journey, whether it is Alzheimer's, vascular dementia, frontotemporal dementia or any other type of dementia.

The study would not have been possible without the study participants, and our knowledge of the experience of dementia is greatly enhanced by their wonderful contributions.

PART 1

Building the Evidence for Spiritual Reminiscence: Research and Theory

1

An Introduction to Spiritual Reminiscence

A critical feature of this study of spiritual reminiscence was exploration of meaning for people as they experience dementia. This chapter provides the rationale for using spiritual reminiscence work with people who have dementia and places the study in the context of current understandings of dementia. It grounds the project in spirituality and, in particular, in the importance of narrative to finding meaning. We begin with story because story is crucial to the formation of human identity, and it is loss of identity that is often most feared in the journey into this disease.

Narrative and understanding of 'self'

There is growing interest in the formation and use of story, and as a result narrative gerontology has become a special interest area within the speciality of gerontology. There are different ways of examining story, and Damasio (2010) brings a neurobiologist's perspective to understanding narrative and the self that is helpful in the context of this project. He describes an autobiographical self that may be overt, 'making up the conscious mind at its grandest and most human' (p.210), but at other times, Damasio writes, the autobiographical self may 'lie dormant, its myriad components waiting their turn to become active' (p.210). In introducing the topic of the autobiographical self, Damasio notes that our autobiographies draw upon our entire life experience as a 'memorized history' that 'describe the most refined among our emotional experiences, namely, those that might qualify as spiritual' (p.210).

Damasio suggests that the maturation of the self may take place 'offscreen' at least to some extent:

...as lived experiences are reconstructed and replayed, whether in conscious reflections or in nonconscious processing, their substance is reassessed and inevitably rearranged, modified minimally or very much in terms of their factual composition and emotional accompaniment. Entities and events acquire new emotional weights during this process. Some frames of the recollection are dropped on the mind's cutting-room floor, others are restored and enhanced, and others still are so deftly combined either by our wants or by the vagaries of chance that they create new scenes that were never shot. That is how, as years pass, our own history is subtly rewritten. That is why facts can acquire a new significance and why the music of memory plays differently today than it did last year. (Damasio 2010, pp.210–211)

An important part of life is assigning meaning to life's events and experiences throughout the life journey. At some points, as Damasio has written, awareness of this process may be more or less conscious than at others. It is likely to be more conscious, for example, as Frankl (1984) has recorded, as we face our own mortality; it may be then that we are able to see the meaning of our lives, perhaps for the first time. Frankl has likened the process of moving from provisional meanings in life to final life meaning as being like the making of a movie. At each event of our lives we shoot the next frame, but these may remain isolated shots through our lives, until we face our own mortality, and then, for the first time, we are able to play the full movie. It is then that we are able to make the connections in our lives, to see the meaning of events that we had once thought were isolated and perhaps meaningless. This may give rise to 'Aha!' experiences; it may even mean a reframing of our life-meaning to take account of our insights into previous life events and our part in them.

Much has been written in recent years of narrative gerontology (Kenyon, Clark and de Vries 2001), of life review, of reminiscence (Gibson 2004; Webster and Haight 2002), of spiritual reminiscence (Morgan 1995, 2003) and of spiritual autobiography (Birren and Cochran 2001). The broad area of reminiscence has gained a great deal of focus and popularity in recent decades. But most of this work was originally done with people who were cognitively competent. In fact, little thought seems to have been given to story and people with dementia. Assumptions seem to have been made that story was only about facts, placing importance on the veracity of the historical record, and the ability to remember was vital to having a story. This goes to the core of human identity, as one's story is linked closely with a sense of identity, and without this, and even more, without being able to articulate one's story, it has often been assumed that there is no story and thus no person.

Narrative and the person with dementia

The matter of story lies at the base of assumptions that if the person has dementia, they are 'no longer there', and a vital part of this assumption is the fact that the person has increasing difficulty in expressing themselves through speech. If they cannot tell their story, it is assumed they have no story. However, this is not necessarily the case, as we have found in the extensive work we have now done with people who have dementia. The need to find meaning is often heightened in importance at critical times of life, for example a life-threatening illness, the diagnosis of dementia, or admission to an aged care facility when experiencing frailty in later life.

And so the question: Is narrative still possible for the person with dementia? An account by a pastoral carer, working in a dementia-specific unit, shows that, even with advanced dementia, narrative, although fractured, may still be present, if given an opportunity to emerge. The incident involved a woman with dementia sitting in a room by herself, in a water-chair; she had been placed in the room on her own because she kept calling out and disturbing others. The pastoral carer went into the room and simply sat with her, just quietly, for half an hour. It was at that point that the woman said: 'In despair, in the chair… Is dull, is horrible, just sitting in this chair… It's not good, could be worse.' This woman, with almost no speech left, was able to articulate her distress when someone sat with her for long enough for her to be able to speak it. Generally within an aged care facility, staff workloads do not allow for staff to be present with a resident for any period of time beyond the essential physical care. It is significant that it was a pastoral carer who went and sat with this woman. It is significant because the central role of the pastoral carer is to be 'present' with others.

The problem is that with dementia, communication skills are progressively lost, and we often cannot expect the story to emerge with the same degree of fluency as it would in a person who is cognitively intact. So is it worth pursuing the possibility of calling forth story in people with dementia? This study has reinforced, for us, the importance of learning skills to call forth the words of these people. We have often been surprised at the ways in which numbers of these people have been able to make their meaning clear, when someone has been willing to be present with them. In subsequent chapters of this book we will provide examples drawn from our research and examples from practice where this has been possible.

It takes patience and time and the ability to be present with the person with dementia for story to begin to emerge. When we began listening to the stories of people with dementia (all in residential care) using in-depth interviews, we not uncommonly initially received responses like 'But I'm only an ordinary person – I don't have a story' (Trevitt and MacKinlay 2006), yet as we gently encouraged the person to speak, the story would often emerge. It is through narrative, the person's life story, that meaning can be found and affirmed. Being present with these people is privileged work, and as we ponder the relationship between the person with dementia and care provider, which this requires, we become aware of the implications and depth of relationship in these interactions. We have become aware that in this process we are actually tapping into the spiritual dimension. Here we are careful to distinguish between the spiritual and religious dimensions. We also need to establish the parameters of what we consider to be the spiritual dimension.

The relationship between religiousness and the spiritual dimension

It is important to put a context on the dimension being discussed. Sometimes religion and spirituality are used interchangeably, while some people declare themselves to be 'spiritual' but not 'religious'. In the context of this work, religion is the term used to describe the practice of a religious faith that includes a community of believers, doctrine and a body of understood religious behaviours and practices. Koenig, McCullough and Larson (2001) distinguish between religion and spirituality through defining religion as an organised system of beliefs, practices, rituals and symbols designed:

(a) to facilitate closeness to the sacred or transcendent (God, higher power, or ultimate truth/reality) and

(b) to foster an understanding of one's relationship and responsibility to others in living together in a community. (p.18)

Second, they define spirituality as:

...the personal quest for understanding answers to ultimate questions about life, about meaning, and about relationship to the sacred or transcendent, which may (or may not) lead to or arise from the development of religious rituals and the formation of community. (p.18)

From the above definitions it can be seen that there is a very close relationship between religion and spiritual, but there are also differences. One of the important differences lies in the fact that the spiritual dimension can be what the individual wants it to be, and can differ markedly from person to person, while religion is more likely to follow a predictable format. One way that helps to see the relationship between religion and spirituality is shown in Figure 1.1.

Figure 1.1 shows that the spiritual dimension is mediated through relationship, environment/creation, the arts and religion. For those who practise a well-functioning religion, each of these four components plays an important part in their religion. Those who do not practise a religious faith fulfil their spirituality through relationship, the whole environment and the arts. However, aspects often considered to be religious, such as symbols and rituals, will likely form a part of the secular person's repertoire as well.

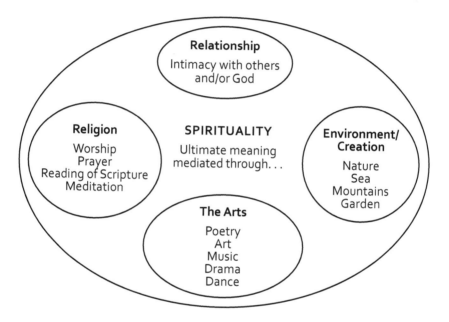

Figure 1.1 *Ways of mediating the spiritual dimension (adapted from MacKinlay 2006)*

Relationship

Humans long for relationship and deep connections with others. Life-meaning for most people is found through relationship. For many this comes through family, life partners, children and, in some cases, deep friendships. In many religious faiths, life-meaning is centred on God. Further, the religious faith is lived within close relationships in the community of the believers. For people of some religious faiths and people of no religious background, life-meaning through relationship with other humans becomes the first priority.

How can relationship be seen as a spiritual focus rather than a psychological focus? There are associations between the two, but the main difference is concerned with degree of relationship; it appears that the spiritual dimension lies more deeply and that it goes to the depths of what it means to be human, to the connections that bring life and hope, even in adversity.

Environment/creation

There is wonder in our world, in our environment, in the whole of the created order. Who has not responded to the beauty of a sunrise, or sunset? Or perhaps responded to the beauty of a flower or the sense of walking in a forest, being by the ocean or being or working in a garden? There is a sense of awe about these connections, something that takes us out of the immediate and transports us to another plane. The natural environment provides connecting points between individuals and communities of different faiths and cultures.

Many humans develop special relationships with animals, and in many ways these connections may be important and life-giving. Two participants in our study said that their most important relationships were with their horses. These were women who lived in rural communities. Environment relates to both the natural and human-made environments, for example responding to the beauty of a Gothic cathedral, a temple or shrines and mosques. The whole of creation and human imagination are part of the continuing process of creation and are rightly included within this sphere.

The arts

Poetry, art, music, drama and dance. All these modes of expression and appreciation help to transport people to another level of being. Sometimes, it is the person with dementia who responds deeply to one of these modes – in a sense of human 'being'. The arts are ways of connecting with symbol and ritual and meaning. We often express the deepest things of life through symbol. Some things are too deep to be just spoken about, but they may be sung, painted, danced or spoken in poetry. Again, that human sense of awe can often be better expressed through the arts.

When language is no longer possible, the arts can provide an important connecting point to others and to otherness. In our deepest times of need – in tragedy, in joy, in love – symbols can connect us with the spiritual and with our God. The arts take humans across faith and cultural barriers to a place where we can connect as humans, in a broader sense of being.

Religion

Religion is a way of connecting with the spiritual. It cannot be separated from the spiritual dimension, or it becomes nothingness. In fact, in a well-functioning religion, it takes in all of the ways of mediating the spiritual: relationship with God and others, responding to the environment, through creation (remembering who we are as part of the whole creation), and of the arts through ritual, liturgy, music, poetry, drama and art. Religion provides the means of worship, community and a structure for the working out of human spirituality. Prayer and meditation connect with ultimate meaning. Good worship should bring a sense of awe, rather than entertainment. Worship is not simply for human enjoyment but is about connecting with the Ultimate, with God.

Meaning in later life: A way into the spiritual dimension

It is well known that many people become more introspective as they grow older. As long back as the 1960s Neugarten (1968) found this in her studies of middle-aged to older adults. Part of this growing introspection is couched in terms of the questions more often being asked by those who are growing older – What is the purpose of my life? Where do I find meaning? and then, perhaps, more urgently, Where do I find meaning now that I am growing older? MacKinlay's (1998, 2001a) work in mapping the spiritual dimension of older adults in an Australian study in the 1990s focused on this aspect of meaning in ageing. This study's participants were independent-living older adults.

This was to be the first of a number of studies that gradually built up a body of knowledge on meaning in later life, first with independent older people, then with frail elderly but cognitively intact people, and finally with people who have dementia. Meaning as an important component of the spiritual dimension was evident in each of these studies. The main modes of data collection for the initial studies of meaning in later life (MacKinlay 2001a) were in-depth interviews of people over the age of 65 years (Minichiello *et al.* 1995). In essence, these interviews focused on the life stories or the narrative of these older people. Interviews that give the opportunity for people to tell *their* story are a valuable way of discovering new knowledge, and the methods chosen to conduct research are important. However, a survey conducted concurrently by MacKinlay using a questionnaire designed by Highfield (1992) with these older people, when analysed using factor analysis, failed to elicit a major theme that was important to these older people in their stories, that is, relationship. This was an important reminder that questionnaires are only as good as the questions used in their construction; the study design for the basis of this book is described further in chapter 3.

It was vital to listen to the words of these older people in seeking to find out more about the spiritual journey of later life (MacKinlay 2001a). In essence, this was a mapping exercise, exploring the spiritual dimension of a sample of older people in Australia. The nature of the initial study led to the choice of qualitative data collection and analysis, as little research had previously examined this area. The data from the in-depth interviews was transcribed from the audio-tapes and analysed by hand, using grounded theory to examine the transcripts for the themes that were important to these people (Glaser 1978; Glaser and Strauss 1967; Morse 1992; Strauss 1987; Strauss and Corbin 1990).

This was a valuable means of developing an understanding of the themes of importance to these people, and allowed the construction of a model of spiritual themes in the lives of the older people in this study, which was the focus of doctoral studies (MacKinlay 1998). From the words and consequent themes of their stories, it was then possible to develop a model of the tasks and process of spiritual development in later life. Obviously, this model could not be generalised, built as it was on the stories of older adults and analysed by qualitative research, but it did provide a starting point from which to examine the spiritual journey of some older people (24 in the in-depth interviews in the first study). This model was subsequently tested in an in-depth study of frail older adults in residential care (20 participants), and then the model was used again and tested against the findings of mixed-methods longitudinal studies of more than 130 people.

A model of the spiritual dimension of ageing and the consequent tasks and process of ageing

There are two models, first the model constructed from the themes of the older people's stories, and then the model of spiritual tasks and process of ageing, drawn from the data of the in-depth stories. The models constructed are discussed in depth in MacKinlay (2001a,b, 2006). A summary of the model is valuable in the context of this book, as it was used as a framework through which to explore and examine meaning in life for the people with dementia. It is therefore important to provide this summary of the model here.

Model of the spiritual themes of ageing

The first model was constructed from the themes of the older people in the original study. The important theme of meaning in life, for the older people living independently, often came through relationships, especially with a life partner, or with adult children, grandchildren and great grandchildren. For frail older people the ultimate of central meaning was more often found through God, however God was perceived by the person. It is noted that in many cases these frail elderly people had lost all significant relationships through death. Central or core meaning, that is, what lay at their hearts, became their motivation for life, and was thus how they responded to all of life.

If what lay at the centre, for instance a satisfying relationship, human or other, was life-giving, then the person was likely to see hope in their lives and to see life as meaningful. They responded to life-meaning through relationship or through worship, music, the arts, or creation and environment. A sense of a loving God at the centre of life became a source of hope, while a sense of a vengeful God might have brought despair. So out of the response to ultimate meaning came four other major themes. These were all continua, first self-sufficiency versus vulnerability; provisional versus final meanings; relationship versus isolation; and hope versus despair. The model of the spiritual themes of ageing is shown in Figure 1.2.

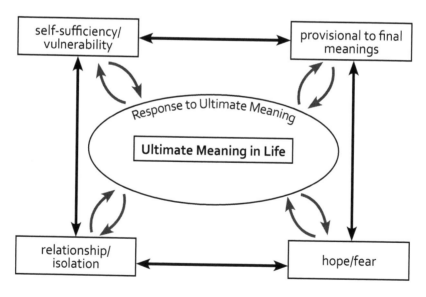

Figure 1.2 *The spiritual themes of ageing*

Model for the spiritual tasks and process of ageing

This model was constructed from the model of the themes, based on the data analysed from the stories of the older people. Thus for the theme of ultimate meaning, the task became to find ultimate meaning. This was often more important for the person who faced their forthcoming death, whether through a terminal illness, or through increasing age and frailty. Some people did not wish to acknowledge their approaching mortality. Response to ultimate meaning was of course related to where that individual found their meaning, and varied greatly from person to person. The theme of self-sufficiency versus vulnerability became the task of self-transcendence or self-forgetting in the presence of loss and disability; the theme of provisional to final meanings became the task to seek out their final life-meaning or purpose; and the theme of relationship versus isolation was to find new intimacies with God and/or others. The final theme, while associated with all other themes, was the theme of hope versus despair. The task is to find hope in the face of loss and disability and coming to terms with meaning and intimacy in later life (see Figure 1.3).

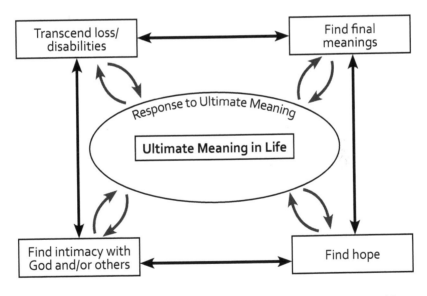

Figure 1.3 *A generic model of the spiritual tasks and process of ageing (from MacKinlay 2006)*

These models have provided valuable frameworks for pastoral and spiritual care with people who are cognitively intact. And it was in this context that they were originally constructed. The beginnings of the models lay with concepts of well ageing, or positive ageing, and of flourishing and resilience in later life. They have provided an important basis for working with older adults who are exploring their lives and purposefully aiming to grow spiritually in their later years. This can be done with older people, one-on-one or in small groups in the community, or in retirement settings. At the time of the original studies, this method of spiritual reminiscence, of linking reminiscence or life review with God's story and the person's story, was not considered by Elizabeth for people with dementia. At least, this was so, until the close and personal experience of working with a person who had dementia. That changed the focus of doing spiritual reminiscence completely; this is discussed in the next section of this chapter.

Personal encounter with dementia: The spiritual journey of Christine and Elizabeth

Sometimes it takes a personal encounter to see a different way of looking at an issue. This happened to Elizabeth, when she first began journeying with Christine Bryden (Boden), after she had been diagnosed with early-onset Alzheimer's, later to be re-diagnosed as frontotemporal dementia. As a nurse, and nurse academic, working particularly with people who have dementia, Elizabeth had a good knowledge of dementia care management. She had thought that she was knowledgeable in person-centred care as well. But her attitudes and knowledge base were about to be challenged at a very profound level. Elizabeth's meeting and involvement with Christine challenged her whole framework of how she saw and how she provided care for people with dementia. Neither her nursing knowledge nor her ministry knowledge had prepared her for the journey that she was to now embark upon. She was about to learn to see the person whole within the experience of dementia. The following is an account of Elizabeth's beginning journey with Christine into dementia.

Christine had asked me to walk the journey into dementia with her, using all of my background of both nurse and priest. I must admit that I was initially apprehensive about how effective this might be. As a nurse I could see the difficulties of journeying in a role of spiritual guide with a person who had dementia.

I asked myself how I might connect with her at a cognitive level, as I had thought this would be really difficult as she gradually lost cognitive function. After all, we so often connect with and relate to people at a cognitive level; it is the way that our societies function. This was the perceived nurse 'management' role. Before I was able to walk with Christine effectively, I had to let go of the need to control the situation. I had to be willing to be vulnerable myself, in this interaction between the person with dementia and the person walking with her. This was a new experience for me.

As we met regularly over the weeks and months, at least fortnightly in that first year or so, I began to learn that it was possible to speak with Christine about dementia; it was no longer the unspoken 'elephant in the room'. Having named it took a great deal of the power of the disease away. Often it is the stigma of a mental illness, or as in this case, the stigma of a brain disease and the myths that surround it, that carries the power to isolate those who have the disease from their loved ones and from those who care for them.

Without that invitation from Christine to walk a journey into dementia with her, I might not have chosen to walk this particular journey. As we continued to meet regularly, I became aware of the fact that what we shared together was too important not to be shared with others. So I suggested to Christine that what we talked about and what we reflected upon would be valuable for others who had dementia. Would it be possible for her to write a book? One of the critical factors in coming to this decision for me was Christine's crucial question: 'Will I lose God as I continue to travel into this disease?' It is always easy to talk about physical ailments or diseases – the person has pneumonia, or has fallen and broken their hip. Of course you would ask, are you getting better, or how is your hip today? (Further discussion of this journey is contained in MacKinlay 2011.)

These questions raised in this journey with Christine are not generally asked in dementia. First, we know the person is unlikely to be getting better, so it is a topic to avoid as at least we will be uncomfortable asking; second, to actually ask about dementia is certainly 'off limits' – or is it?

Naming dementia

Why can't we speak of dementia to those who have it? The stigma of this disease (stigma is dealt with further in chapters 2 and 4) is seen in the following comment of a daughter who did not wish her mother, who had dementia, to take part in our research project. She said: 'It will be fine for Mum to take part, as long as you don't mention dementia – Mum doesn't know she has dementia' (this woman was in residential aged care due to her dementia). The mother may well have known that she had dementia, but mother and daughter were unable to name it and speak of it together. This is an all too common occurrence.

It is still too hard to speak of dementia. Just as it seems, as we have overcome our reluctance to speak of other taboo subjects, of cancer, of sex and, to some extent, of death and dying, so we need to learn at all levels of society to speak of dementia, with each other and those who live with it. What was so powerful for Elizabeth in beginning to walk this journey with Christine was to realise that they could speak of dementia, and this took away so much of the power of the disease. Naming it enabled them to talk of it openly. How did it feel? Early after her diagnosis, Christine became depressed. At first she felt completely isolated, but at some point she sensed that God was with her in this blackness that she experienced. She found it helpful to reflect on this and to affirm her faith in this journey that had only just begun. Being able to talk about her emotions and her spiritual being at this time was helpful to her. Christine's journey is more thoroughly dealt with in her two books *Who Will I Be When I Die?* (Boden 1998) and *Dancing with Dementia* (Bryden 2005).

As Christine and Elizabeth journeyed together, Christine spoke of the importance to her of being able to find meaning in the experience of this disease. Without meaning, there is no hope. It was this meaning that she struggled to find. This struck a key for Elizabeth and the need to learn more about how to communicate with and connect with people who have dementia. Elizabeth was learning much from Christine, but, she had to ask, was this just a very special case? Could other people also experience dementia in similar ways to Christine? After all, she was well educated, and she had a high IQ before she was diagnosed with dementia; perhaps she was an isolated case. So an important question began to take shape for Elizabeth – could other people also benefit from talking about dementia; could quality of life be improved by opening up the conversation for people with dementia, their loved ones and carers? A whole theory about dementia could not be built just on the basis of a sample of one; it was important to look further.

This was an important step towards further research to develop care and communication strategies for people with dementia. Of course, the conversation concerns two parties, those who have dementia and those who travel the journey with them – their loved ones and carers. In our work to date, we have focused on people with dementia; others have focused on the carers of people with dementia. Both aspects are important; however, it seemed to us, as we set out to embark on this particular direction of study, that it was particularly urgent to map out the possibilities for connecting with the people who have dementia themselves.

Spirituality and dementia

We have looked briefly at narrative or story in later life and its place in coming to final life-meanings; we have also noted the possibilities of using story with people who have dementia, to assist them in finding meaning. It is valuable as well to examine the spiritual dimension in the context of dementia. Swinton (2008) has made the important connection between dementia as a disease of the brain, with biological consequences for memory, intellect and rationality, and dementia as a culturally defined disease. Fear of dementia remains real in our communities; a future diagnosis of dementia was given as a reason to contemplate suicide by one participant in Elizabeth's initial studies in the mid-1990s – there is no reason to assume that this woman's fear of getting dementia is either isolated or that attitudes have changed since then. In fact 70 per cent of the group of independent living older people in that study (MacKinlay 2001a), when asked if they had any fear for the future, mentioned dementia as a fear.

In a very important sense, the way into connecting with people who have dementia is not through cognitive means, but through the emotional and spiritual means of connecting with others. A small book picked up by chance – *Dementia: Pastoral Theology and Pastoral Care* – notes that 'gentle neglect of people with dementia is not a worthy pastoral strategy for the church – and yet this is often the case in practice' (Saunders 2002, p.21). Within residential aged care facilities, sometimes people will say that it is of no value to include those with dementia in church services 'because they would not know what is going on'. Yet, as is also now widely known and acknowledged, people with dementia, even advanced dementia, can and do respond to spiritual and emotional experiences.

Oliver Sacks (1985) published some of the earliest examples of the unexpected responses and connections made by people with dementia and other neurological conditions to religious and spiritual experiences. A classic example was the story of 'Jimmy', a man with Korsakoff's syndrome who seemed to have no cognitive function at all. Jimmy seemed not to be able to hold a thought in his mind. Sacks had asked the Sisters who cared for him (1985, p.36): 'Do you think he has a soul?' They were outraged by this question and responded: 'Watch Jimmy in chapel…and judge for yourself.' Sacks did just that, and reported his amazement at the difference he witnessed there. There he saw Jimmy 'absorbed in an act, an act of his whole being, which carried feeling and meaning in an organic continuity and unity'. This experience brought the words of Luria to Sacks' mind as he wrote (Sacks 1985, p.36): 'A man does not consist of memory alone. He has feeling, will, sensibility, moral being…it is here…you may touch him and see a profound change.'

Sacks (1985) found then that Jimmy did not just respond in the chapel, but was also able to respond to music and art, and he started working in the garden. Importantly, Sacks noted that while Jimmy could be 'held' for a brief time in a puzzle or game, he would 'fall apart' as soon as these activities were finished. However, in contrast, he could be held in art or music, or the chapel or garden, and that 'mood' would persist for a time, and they would see a peace in him, rarely ever seen otherwise. We suspect that this may be something of what we have encountered through the process of spiritual reminiscence. Sacks completes this story of Jimmy with the following reflection, which is of great significance for what we are attempting to do in the search for meaning and connection for people who live with dementia. Sacks wrote:

> I had wondered when I first met him, if he [Jimmy] were not condemned to a sort of 'Humean' froth, a meaningless fluttering on the surface of life, and whether there was any way of transcending the incoherence of his Humean disease. Empirical science told me there was not – but empirical science, empiricism, takes no account of the soul, no account of what constitutes and determines personal being. Perhaps there is a philosophical as well as a clinical lesson here: that in Korsakov's, or dementia, or other such catastrophes, however great the organic damage and Humean dissolution, there remains the undiminished possibility of reintegration by art, by communion, by touching the human spirit: and this can be preserved in what seems at first a hopeless state of neurological devastation. (Sacks 1985, pp.37–38)

Although Sacks wrote this in the 1980s, we still have a long way to go in changing attitudes and views of dementia that seem to be prevalent in some areas of the wider community and indeed in at least some aged care settings.

In the book *Ageing, Spirituality and Disability* (MacKinlay 2008) Elizabeth wrote of the person with profound dementia who could neither speak nor move, who when diagnosed with cancer had pastoral and religious services reinstated into his routine at home. His widow wrote of the wonder of seeing her husband move his hand, a hand that had not moved for some considerable time, to take the bread as he received Communion. This had previously been denied to him on the basis of his dementia.

From time to time, we still hear of examples of care providers excluding people with dementia from services of worship and other engagement with others on the basis of their cognitive function.

Spiritual reminiscence and its application in dementia

Spiritual reminiscence is a particular way of communication that acknowledges the person as a spiritual being and seeks to engage the person in a more meaningful and personal way. Spiritual reminiscence as we have developed and applied it, especially in working with people who have dementia, has been through the model of the spiritual tasks and process of ageing, as outlined earlier in this chapter.

Summary

In this first chapter, the topics of narrative and of spirituality in later life and their place in dementia have been outlined. Recent scholarship in the fields of spirituality and ageing has formed the background and rationale for the main studies that provided the reason for the work and this book. As the importance of narrative in later life and in dementia was highlighted, story has been explored as a means of tapping into aspects of meaning for the person who has dementia.

A model of the spiritual tasks and process of ageing has been briefly described, setting the scene for the study and book. The book focuses on a particular kind of reminiscence, that of spiritual reminiscence, that seeks to connect with meaning for the person who has dementia. The relationship between spirituality and religion has also been explored. It is acknowledged that the focus of this book is on the person with dementia, although we most definitely acknowledge the vital importance of the relationship of the person with dementia and those who accompany that person on their journey into this disease. Care providers will find many examples to guide their practice in working with spiritual reminiscence for people with dementia.

2

Current Understandings of Dementia and Implications for Care

Dementia is a term that encompasses many different diseases and a variety of symptoms. When we generally think of dementia we think of memory loss. But the memory loss is a small (though for many a significant) part of the changes that occur. There are also many different behavioural changes that can have a great impact on quality of life for the person with dementia and for their friends and relatives. Many people with dementia require long-term care as their condition gradually worsens. This chapter will examine the issues that are most frequently associated with dementia. We will describe the different types of dementia and their prevalence; the impact of a diagnosis of dementia and the stigma that is attached to this diagnosis; and the types of treatments available – biomedical, psychosocial and spiritual.

The current picture of dementia – prevalence and incidence

The number of people with dementia is presented in two ways – by prevalence and incidence. A prevalence survey provides a snapshot of the number of people with dementia at any one time. This includes people who have been diagnosed for years or those recently diagnosed. The number of people with dementia is then estimated as a proportion of the total population. Incidence, on the other hand, is the process of taking a population of people and tracking them over the long term as they age and identifying those who develop dementia. Both these measures are very important and allow for both short-term and long-term planning. As a population ages there can be the expectation that the numbers of those with dementia in that population will increase – prevalence. However, what is possibly even more important is whether the incidence is increasing – are more people in a population developing dementia?

The most comprehensive world-wide survey of dementia prevalence was published in 2005 (Ferri *et al.*). It was estimated that in 2005 world-wide there were 24 million people with dementia and that this was expected to double every 20 years to 42 million by 2020 and 81 million by 2040. This progression assumed that there would be no changes in mortality and no effective treatments. What is most interesting from this survey is that data from South America, Africa and the old USSR were either very patchy or non-existent. At that time it was estimated that countries with the greatest number of people with dementia were China (5.0 million), the European Union (5.0 million), the USA (2.9 million), India (1.5 million), Japan (1.1 million), Russia (1.1 million) and Indonesia (1.0 million) (Ferri *et al.* 2005). The authors do say, however, that some of these data should be treated with caution because of the paucity of quality epidemiological data.

In terms of incidence, it is shown that as the population ages the likelihood of developing dementia increases exponentially. Annual incidence rates reported by the EURODEM meta-analysis suggest that the average disease duration is four years. Clinical studies, however, indicate that this is nearer five to seven years, and with good clinical care this can be longer. Dementia is certainly a more common disease nowadays than 50 to 100 years ago, but this is because there is a general trend towards an ageing population. Although dementia is not a normal ageing change, ageing is a risk factor for dementia. So, despite the increase in numbers of people with dementia, there is no evidence that it is becoming more prevalent (Alzheimer's Disease International 2008).

In Australia, recent data from Access Economics (2009) suggests that in 2009 there were 245,400 people with dementia, with expectations that this will rise to around 1.13 million by 2050. The incidence is expected to increase from 69,600 new cases in 2009 to 385,000 new cases in 2050. As people age, the expectation that they could develop dementia also rises. At age 70–74 years there is a 3.5 per cent chance of developing dementia. By the age of 85 years this has risen to a 21.1 per cent chance (Access Economics 2009). What is striking from this data is that 79 per cent of those over 85 will *not* develop dementia – the vast majority will remain cognitively capable until they die – a fact we tend to forget when we examine dementia data. Although dementia is largely a disease of older people, about 2 per cent of new dementia diagnoses are for people under the age of 65 (Alzheimer's Disease International 2008). As the number of people with dementia increases, there will be a significant impact on provision of care for these people. Access Economics (2009) has summarised the health and financial impact:

- Dementia is the leading single cause of disability in older Australians (aged 65 years or older) and is responsible for one year in every six years of disability burden for this group.

- It is one of the fastest growing sources of major disease burden, overtaking coronary heart disease in its total well-being cost by 2023.

- Dementia will become the third greatest source of health and residential aged care spending within about two decades. These costs alone will be around 1 per cent of GDP.

- By the 2060s, spending on dementia is set to outstrip that of any other health condition. It is projected to be AU$83 billion and will represent around 11 per cent of the entire health and residential aged care sector spending.

(Access Economics 2009)

In the USA there is a similar picture for dementia. The summary for the USA looks like this:

- More than five million Americans are believed to have Alzheimer's disease and, by 2050, the number could increase to over 15 million.

- The national cost of Alzheimer's disease (in people over 65 years old) was $US183 billion in 2011; by 2050 it will be $US1 trillion.

- By 2048, 1 in 45 people may be living with Alzheimer's disease.

- Approximately five per cent of all cases of Alzheimer's disease are believed to be familial (hereditary). In familial cases, often called early-onset Alzheimer's disease, symptoms typically appear within the age range of 30–60 years.

- The lifetime risk of Alzheimer's disease among those who reach the age of 65 is approximately 1 in 5 for women and 1 in 10 among men.

- Approximately 70 per cent of Alzheimer's disease patients receive care at home.

- In terms of healthcare expenses and lost wages of both patients and their caregivers, the cost of Alzheimer's disease nationwide is estimated at $US100 billion per year.

(Alzheimer's Disease Research 2011)

And to finish – the story for the UK:

- There are currently 750,000 people with dementia in the UK.

- There are over 16,000 younger people with dementia in the UK.

- There will be over a million people with dementia by 2021.

- Two thirds of people with dementia are women.

- The proportion of people with dementia doubles for every five-year age group.

- Delaying the onset of dementia by five years would reduce deaths directly attributable to dementia by 30,000 a year.

- The financial cost of dementia to the UK is over £20 billion a year.

- Family carers of people with dementia save the UK over £6 billion a year.

- Sixty-four per cent of people living in care homes have a form of dementia.

- Two thirds of people with dementia live in the community while one third live in a care home.

(Alzheimer's Society 2011)

What can be seen from the summaries of each of these countries is that there is a growing concern about the financial impact of dementia in a society. There is less emphasis on the individual impact and the care for those with dementia. All the rhetoric appears so negative – what are the ways to try to approach this in a more positive and sympathetic light?

Biomedical understandings of dementia

Although we tend to speak about dementia as a disease, the term refers to a symptom of a number of different diseases. The types of behaviours we see in people with dementia include but are not limited to: paranoid and delusional ideation; hallucinations; activity disturbances; aggression and irritability; diurnal rhythm disturbance; depression; apathy; euphoria; eating disturbances; and anxiety phobias (Chiu *et al.* 2006).

Alzheimer's disease is the most common of the dementias – and we frequently use the term dementia and Alzheimer's interchangeably – but there are many different types of dementia. These dementias are differentiated by their presentation, the person's previous medical history and often by the types of behaviours that are the most prevalent. Some, for example Alzheimer's disease, are not fully diagnosed until after death, but improved diagnostic techniques are allowing an early and definitive diagnosis in many cases (Ballard *et al.* 2011).

The other most common types of dementia include vascular dementia, frontotemporal dementia, Parkinson's dementia, Lewy body dementia and mild cognitive impairment. Knowing the type of dementia is useful when planning care. Each type tends to manifest itself in slightly different ways – although many of the primary features of memory loss, confusion, hallucinations and gradual decrease of social functioning remain the same. It can be helpful for carers though to be aware of some of the differences in the different types. For example, those with Alzheimer's tend to have less depression than those with vascular dementia; frontotemporal dementia causes more verbal outbursts and inappropriate activities; and paranoid delusions and hallucinations are more common in dementia with Lewy bodies (Chiu *et al.* 2006). Those with Parkinson's dementia tend to have impaired visuospatial functioning, hallucinations and paranoia (Emre *et al.* 2007). It is important to have an understanding of these different types of behaviours because it is often an exacerbation of these that leads to the person requiring long-term care.

Alzheimer's disease

Alzheimer's disease is named after Alois Alzheimer, who had noted specific behavioural changes in one of his patients. His 51-year-old patient presented with a five-year history of confusion, hallucinations, severe cognitive impairment and poor social functioning. Autopsy showed the characteristic amyloid plaques and neurofibrillary tangles that we now associate with Alzheimer's disease (Ferri *et al.* 2005). Alzheimer's disease is the most common type of dementia and the one we hear most about. On average, patients with Alzheimer's disease live for eight to ten years after diagnosis, but this fatal disease can last as long as 20 years, or as little as three to four years if the patient is over 80 years old when diagnosed (Alzheimer's Disease Research 2011).

There are a number of characteristic behaviours that people can notice when developing dementia. We all hear about confusion and memory loss, but other aspects of daily life can also be affected. People may experience mood swings, become less interested in life, or become depressed or anxious. Simple everyday tasks may become more difficult – things such as preparing a meal, setting the table, getting dressed, shopping or dealing with money. Because of these difficulties, people find it becomes harder to take care of themselves. We talk about some communication issues in chapter 12, but commonly people may struggle to complete sentences or find the correct word. As the disease progresses, people become frail and increasingly dependent.

Vascular dementia

Vascular dementia is the next most common dementia. It arises predominantly from the concept of arteriosclerotic dementia characterised by areas of ischaemia (tissue death) caused by numerous mini-strokes or hardening of the cerebral arteries. However, there is increasing evidence that there is considerable overlap between Alzheimer's disease and vascular dementia and that one enhances and encourages the other (Iadecola 2010; Viswanathan, Rocca and Tzourio 2009). Evidence shows that reducing cardiovascular risk factors such as hypertension, stroke and diabetes, and increasing exercise and improving diet, act to reduce the incidence of both vascular and Alzheimer's disease (Iadecola 2010). Many of the behaviours of vascular dementia are similar to Alzheimer's disease – although the particular behaviour may be more associated with the area of the brain affected by ischaemia. Also, those with vascular dementia can sometimes experience plateaus in the progression of the disease, unlike a steadier loss seen in Alzheimer's.

Frontotemporal dementia

Frontotemporal dementia (FTD) refers to a group of disorders that are characterised by neurodegeneration of the prefrontal and anterior temporal lobes. The earliest recognised of these was Pick's disease, described by Arnold Pick in 1892. He described a number of language and behavioural difficulties that have come to be recognised as part of FTD (Lipton and Boxer 2009). Other diseases associated with these areas of the brain are progressive aphasia and semantic dementia. Some patients have a mixed clinical picture of FTD, semantic dementia and progressive aphasia. Age at onset is generally between 45 and 65 years. The median duration of the illness from diagnosis to death is between 6 and 8 years, with a range of 2–20 years (Neary, Snowden and Mann 2005).

The behavioural changes seen in FTD are different to those seen in Alzheimer's disease and vascular dementia. Early in the disease progress there is a decline in interpersonal conduct, regulation of personal conduct, emotional blunting and loss of insight. Other behaviours include eating to excess, disinhibition, hoarding and sometimes criminal behaviours such as stalking and shoplifting (Lipton and Boxer 2009). Also, executive functions such as planning, judgement, problem solving and attention are all affected. By contrast, spatial skills, elementary visual perception and memory are well preserved. Compared with those with Alzheimer's disease, people with FTD can negotiate their environment with ease (Neary *et al.* 2005). There has been no identified treatment for FTD, but the use of anti-depressants can be useful in dealing with the behavioural issues (Lipton and Boxer 2009).

Parkinson's dementia

Parkinson's disease (PD) is the second most common neurodegenerative disease and affects about 1 per cent of the population over 60 years of age (Edison *et al.* 2008). People who have been diagnosed with PD have about a 30 per cent chance of developing dementia. PD occurs when there is a loss of dopamine in the substantia nigra area of the brain and is characterised by bradykinesia (slow movements), stiffness and rigidity. Most of these symptoms can be ameliorated with medication, but this does not prevent dementia occurring (Hely *et al.* 2008). People with PD are more likely to develop dementia as they age and as the length of time they have had PD increases, especially if they have the more severe form of the disease (Emre *et al.* 2007). The types of symptoms seen in dementia associated with PD include loss of short-term recall and visuospatial and executive functions, personality and behavioural changes, hallucinations and confusion (Edison *et al.* 2008).

Lewy body dementia

Lewy body dementia has come to be recognised as separate from other forms of dementia since the 1980s. The characteristic Lewy bodies are found in up to 40 per cent of brains of elderly patients with dementia at post-mortem. It is often difficult to diagnose but does have some specific features (Tarawneh and Galvin 2009). These include: fluctuations in cognition with pronounced variations in alertness and attention; recurrent hallucinations that are detailed and well formed; and spontaneous features of Parkinsonism (McKeith *et al.* cited in Edison *et al.* 2008). People with Lewy body dementia have better memory-preservation skills than those with Alzheimer's disease, but they have marked visuospatial and visuoperceptual problems. This often makes it difficult for them to navigate around their house or move out of bed or a chair (Tarawneh and Galvin 2009). Fluctuations in cognition are also seen in between 15 and 80 per cent of cases.

Mild cognitive impairment

Mild cognitive impairment (MCI) is described as the grey zone between normal cognitive ageing and early dementia. Those with MCI have memory impairment greater than what you would expect for their age but do not meet the commonly accepted criteria for a diagnosis of dementia. So, it is separate from dementia, in which cognitive deficits are more severe and widespread. However, MCI with memory complaints and deficits (amnesic mild cognitive impairment) has a high risk of progression to dementia, particularly of the Alzheimer type, although some have progression to FTD or Lewy body dementia (Geda, Negash and Petersen 2009). The criteria identifying MCI are: a memory complaint usually corroborated by an informant; objective memory impairment for age; essentially preserved general cognitive function; largely intact functional activities; and not demented (Petersen 2004).

It has also been reported that depression (measured using the Geriatric Depression Scale) more than doubled the risk of transition from normal ageing to incident MCI. Four hypotheses were proposed to account for this progression: (1) that depression leads to MCI via neurological pathways; (2) there is a shared risk factor between depression and MCI; (3) that someone experiencing memory loss becomes depressed; and (4) there is an increased susceptibility for MCI following depression. Each of these possibilities is being further explored (Geda *et al.* 2009). Because of the incidence of depression and MCI, depression in older adults needs to be recognised and appropriately treated (Chertkow *et al.* 2008). There have been a number of treatments proposed to help reduce the progression into dementia from MCI. These include medications, exercise, diet and cognitive training. There have been mixed results from these interventions, but there is consensus that treatment of any underlying conditions, including depression, can help the progression of MCI (Chertkow *et al.* 2008).

The effects of dementia on individuals and families

'When Milton's Satan stood in the pit of hell and raged at heaven, he was merely a trifle miffed compared to how I felt on that day.' This was the reaction of bestselling author Terry Pratchett on being diagnosed with Alzheimer's disease.

The diagnosis of dementia can have a huge impact on the person diagnosed and all of his or her friends and relatives. Although we might all go around bemoaning our lack of memory for simple things like car keys and handbags, once a diagnosis of dementia is made each of these admissions seems to be another nail into the coffin of deterioration. For a younger person, their whole life course will be affected. Think back to Christine's story and the impact the diagnosis had on her family and friends and her career. Jim Mann clearly articulates the impact the diagnosis has had on his life. He mentions the stigma he felt and how he became determined to speak up on behalf of those with dementia and the importance of trying to make a difference. In the preface to a recent book he writes:

> We are not all victims. We have a life worth living. While it may not be the life we choose it is what we have... So you know what? We are going to make it ours. And we are going to make it worthwhile. (Bartlett and O'Connor 2010, p.*xi*)

So what is the impact? Earlier in this chapter we examined the impact of dementia on the population and the economy, but how does this translate to the individual concerned? Terry Pratchett has described his despair upon his diagnosis, his subsequent depression and now his plans for his future death – under his control. Each person diagnosed with dementia will have a different response to that diagnosis and a different response to the disease itself. It has been suggested that primary caregivers are reluctant to make a diagnosis of dementia. This is for a number of reasons, including: the possibility of stigma; wanting to protect a person from a difficult diagnosis; lack of confidence in making the diagnosis; or attributing memory loss to the normal ageing process. Families also help to protect the person – by surreptitiously taking over tasks and social roles. There is now a consensus favouring early diagnosis so that treatments that could delay the onset of severe symptoms can be instituted (Iliffe *et al.* 2009). Early diagnosis also allows the person with dementia to make important decisions about their life while they have the cognitive capacity to do so. In many cases this also includes making an advance directive for their future health care (Ballard *et al.* 2011).

Stigma of dementia

It can be seen from conversations with those with dementia that there is a stigma about the dementia diagnosis. This seems strange given that there is nothing that people can do in the majority of cases to have prevented the onset of the disease. It is not like obesity or smoking, where we might think that people had contributed to their ill health. So what is it that makes people reluctant to tell others? Jim Mann describes how he first told someone – how he admitted to having dementia and then felt liberated and determined to forward the cause of those with dementia for as long as he could (Bartlett and O'Connor 2010). Christine Bryden (Boden) has also described the stigma she felt at the diagnosis.

Being diagnosed with dementia has a double impact – society places high value on youth and cognitive attainment – which leads to prejudice. Brooker (2004) describes this as dementia-ism. It is related to all the other –isms, such as ageism, sexism and racism, but also exists on its own. This discrimination can be seen in the provision of services, resource allocation, research funding, media coverage, policy provisions, professional status and training. Additionally, as dementia is associated with mental health conditions, it is a ready candidate for stigmatisation of the person and, by association, for carers and health professionals who care for them – reinforcing the existing societal prejudices towards ageing. Goffman was the first to study stigma and its effects on people; he defined stigma 'as a sign or mark that designates the possessor as "spoiled" and therefore as less valued than "normal" people' (Goffman in Werner and Heinik 2008, p.92). Goffman wrote:

> Stigma is an illuminating excursion into the situation of persons who are unable to conform to standards that society calls normal. Disqualified from full social acceptance, they are stigmatized individuals... Their image of themselves must daily confront and be affronted by the image which others reflect back to them. (Goffman 1963, p.137)

The inability to speak about dementia is a sign of the stigma of this condition. As we see from the comments by Jim Mann and Christine above, it is very difficult for those recently diagnosed to speak of their dementia. In this study, we found that relatives were reluctant to include their loved ones in a 'dementia study' – even though they were in residential care because of their dementia. In an earlier study it was found that 70 per cent of independent older people feared developing dementia. This finding emerged from in-depth interviews in which dementia was not mentioned; the question asked of participants was simply: 'Do you have any fears for the future?' (MacKinlay 1998).

Perhaps the greatest stigma of dementia is the societal notion of 'living death' or of having no further functions to fulfil – of being a 'non-person' or having no value. Behuniak (2011) uses the metaphor of 'zombie' to describe how society seems to view those with dementia – those who are the living dead – constrained by their disease with no sense of self remaining. She examined the literature related to terms that could be associated with the concept of zombie, especially through the milieu of film; she noted that 'zombie' is something that has not only stigma, but is hated and viewed with disgust and fear. This is reinforced by books – there have been a number of publications which characterise Alzheimer's disease and dementia as a living death, for example Robert Woods' *Alzheimer's Disease: Coping with a Living Death* (1989). This social construction, Behuniak contends, was initiated by the biomedical approach to dementia – the person became a body that needed to be managed rather than a person to be cared for and valued.

As we have already mentioned, older people are already discriminated against, with negative stereotypes often predominating within society. Add to this the prevalence of dementia in older age, and the discrimination and stigma become even greater. Corrigan *et al.* (2005) have compared the function of a public health versus social justice approach to reduction of stigma, noting that often a public health approach of education simply shifts the focus off the mental illness, in this case dementia as a mental health problem, to a biological problem of brain disease instead. This may not actually be effective in dealing with the stigma, but instead assist in the development of yet a different stigma, in which the stigmatised person is still blamed for their condition, but for different reasons. The social construction of dementia is a vitally important aspect to consider and forms the main focus of this project.

Milne (2010) has outlined multiple modes of intervention to prevent and overcome stigma. Among these are policy changes, such as the national priorities in numbers of countries now to alleviate the stigma of dementia. She offers the profiling of highly visible people who have dementia and examples of effective lives of those living with it; however, this may become counterproductive as often these people themselves become stigmatised when publicly associated with dementia. Milne rightly endorses an increased range and quality of resources for dementia care, while she notes staff and carer education, with increasing job satisfaction, being key elements of this process. Further, she says that stigma itself needs to be actively attacked. The word 'attack' is frequently used in association with this disease. Milne also lists research as a way forward; the type of research is important, as the approach will need not only research that seeks for cure of dementia, but also considers the person who has dementia and their life experience.

The language used frequently around dementia also highlights the way we view it. George (2010) describes how we view dementia as a 'battle', in how it 'attacks' or 'strikes us down'. The terminology used has a powerful message of war against dementia. He also describes how those with dementia experience 'social death' or 'living death' and that carers experience the 'burden of care'. Ageing is viewed by policy makers as a 'crisis'. Each of these terms reinforces the way we as a society view dementia and ageing.

He contends that the language we use is a very powerful way to provide an extremely negative view of dementia. It may be more effective to think about 'postponement' rather than 'cure'; to remove the stigma of both ageing and dementia and seek the positives from the situation. Instead of concentrating on the 'burden' of caring, look for the joys, sharing, compassion, forgiveness and reconciliation to be gained from caring. To celebrate the progress in public health that ensures a larger population of older people who provide many strengths, talents and wisdom, he provides a very powerful message to counteract the stigma of dementia and ageing via semantics (George 2010). In this book, we endeavour to present some of the actual words of people who have dementia that might broaden this life experience, to include laughter, joy, love and peace, as well as struggle, despair and burnout.

Where most emphasis has been given to promoting personhood among people with dementia to overcome stigma and discrimination, Bartlett and O'Connor (2007) hypothesise that a wider lens is needed to support people with dementia being treated equally to any other persons. They suggest the lens of citizenship as a possible way forward, before critiquing that too as problematic for those with severe dementia. We have found in recent research that in practice the concept of person-centred care does not always translate into reality of care.

Using spiritual reminiscence for people with dementia helps these people to find meaning and goes some way towards addressing just one aspect of this condition. Its contribution towards lowering stigma is to the people who have dementia, in affirming them as people of worth, to their families, as they see changes in their loved ones, and for care providers, who may see the life that is possible among these people.

Biomedical approaches to care

Much of the emphasis on biomedical care has been in finding genetic markers (for Alzheimer's disease), trialling medications that interfere with the pathological changes (again of Alzheimer's disease) and prescribing medications that will impact on the types of behaviours seen in people with dementia. While these approaches may in the long term have a significant impact on the prevalence of Alzheimer's disease, they are mostly concerned with behaviours of dementia rather than with the person with dementia.

Medications have been used widely to manage some of the distressing behaviours in dementia. A recent meta-analysis describes the types and uses of various medications for Alzheimer's disease (Ballard *et al.* 2011). Once diagnosis is made there needs to be a careful assessment of existing medication use – poly-pharmacy can lead to a number of cognitive and physical complications. There are a number of medications used to help with dementia – if you work in an aged care setting or with older adults you will probably recognise many of the names of these. Cholinesterase inhibitors (such as donepezil and rivastigmine) have been used to help improve cognitive function in the short term; however, outcomes are difficult to measure. There is some reported improvement in apathy and social interaction, which impacts favourably on families, but again it is difficult to quantify these within the constraints of a clinical trial (Ballard *et al.* 2011). Other commonly used medications are antipsychotics – used predominantly to control symptoms such as agitation, aggression and psychosis. These include risperidone, olanzapine and aripiprazole. Benefits can be only moderate but side effects are considerable and include sedation, Parkinsonism, chest infections, ankle oedema and increased risk of stroke and death. Potential risks and benefits always need to be considered (Ballard *et al.* 2011). Bird (2002) wrote of his distress when a resident was medicated because of aggression, became heavily sedated and died in a short time – when behaviour modification techniques for staff may have solved the problem.

There is much ongoing research into specific medications that specifically target the physiological changes in Alzheimer's disease; and there are ongoing clinical trials to test the effectiveness of these interventions (Ballard *et al.* 2011). But such current research into dementia causes and treatments will not avail the present and immediate future cohort of those with dementia. Until the 'magic cure' is found – if ever – psychosocial care will remain very important.

While research into medication for dementia remains inconclusive, various risk factors that could lead to a higher incidence of dementia have been examined. There is a large amount of data about non-modifiable risk factors such as age, genetics and head injury. Other risk factors are modifiable, and meta-analysis provides evidence that cognitive reserve (combination of education, occupation and mental activities), exercise, mid-life obesity, alcohol intake and smoking are the most important modifiable risk factors (Ballard *et al.* 2011). A number of treatable diseases are also associated with a higher incidence of dementia – these include stroke, diabetes, mid-life hypertension and mid-life hypercholesterolaemia. Prevention of dementia is probably part of a more widely accepted push to a healthier lifestyle with an emphasis on increased exercise (Ballard *et al.* 2011).

Psychosocial approaches to care

During the last 20–30 years there have been many new ways of caring for those with dementia. We have moved from reality orientation to validation; from management of individual behaviours to a process of person-centred care and dementia care mapping; and to reminiscence therapy and spiritual reminiscence. There are also many activities designed to improve the quality of life such as art and music therapy.

Reality orientation and validation

In the 1960s it was believed that the treatment of those with dementia included 'keeping them up to date' (Taulbee and Folsom 1966). The process included orienting the person to their surroundings including time, place, person and things. There was an assumption that the disoriented person only needed frequent reminding to help them to return to the present. This approach is advantageous for those with temporary delirium – it can help to orient them to reality. However, for those with dementia, reality orientation can contradict their own reality and lead to frustration and anxiety. It can lead to people always been told that they are incorrect, that their home and family is no longer around them or that their husband/wife has passed away. For many people, hearing these things over again can surface anxieties and fears and reduce self-esteem.

Validation, on the other hand, reinforces where the person is now – it is about tapping into the reality for that person, not testing them on the time and place. It can help to reduce anxiety and reduce conflict. Carers may feel that not telling the truth about a situation is not correct and that people with dementia should accept reality, but this is about putting the carer's needs first. As Kitwood maintains, dementia care is about the needs of the person with dementia.

Both these approaches to care have their place. Allowing a person to be surrounded with personal objects from their reality can help as triggers to conversations and expressing memories. However, for many older people with dementia who live in aged care facilities, knowing what day of the week it is or who the Prime Minister (or President) is has little value.

Person-centred care

The term 'person-centred care' was developed in the early 1990s by Tom Kitwood as part of the Bradford Dementia Research Group. He was frustrated by the biomedical paradigm that suggested that the person with dementia was a set of behaviours to manage until the person died. If you are just managing behaviours then there is no need to interact in a meaningful way. He also contended that much of what happens in later life is socially constructed – that physical and psychosocial changes as we get older are more a response to the way we see ourselves as we grow older, and the way others see us. Therefore, if we changed our attitudes and approach to those with dementia, then in turn their response would also change. He used the philosophy of Carl Rogers to examine the concept of 'self' as the basis of his stance. He used the term 'person-centred care' to bring together ideas that emphasise communication and relationships (Brooker 2004, p.215).

Kitwood argued that early dementia care concentrated on the 'problem' of those with dementia. It did not consider the issues surrounding the person with dementia. He proposed that there was an 'us' and 'them' and that 'they' had the problem. In order for 'them' to get over the problem, we had to learn how to care for them and manage their challenging behaviours. In fact, he said that perhaps we were the problem, that perhaps those with dementia were more 'authentic' about what they were feeling and doing – living in the past; and being dependent – whereas we 'normal' people were labouring under the illusion of individualism – finding it difficult to live in the present because of regrets from the past and having fears about the future (Kitwood and Bredin 1992). The loss of personhood came about because of the social and care setting surrounding the person with dementia. Personhood is reflected and reinforced by our social surroundings – it has an ethical status; to be a person is to have a place in society and be worthy of respect. 'It is a standing or status that is bestowed upon one human being, by others, in the context of relationship and social being. It implies recognition, respect and trust' (Kitwood 1997, p.8). By connotation, loss of personhood results in loss of a place in society and consequent loss of respect (Kitwood and Bredin 1992). Person-centred care is based on and came out of this concept of personhood.

Person-centred care has become a 'motherhood statement'. In any documents relating to aged care, person-centred care is discussed. After all, who would disagree with providing care that meets the individual needs of residents? However, in many cases, the complete approach to person-centred care has not been achieved. Kitwood described ten types of behaviours from carers that undermine person-centred care and reinforce the loss of self and respect for those with dementia. He labelled these as 'malignant social psychology'; they include: treachery, disempowerment, infantilisation, condemnation, intimidation, stigmatisation, banishment and objectification (Kitwood 1993). He shifted the emphasis and responsibility for 'difficult behaviours' firmly away from the person with dementia and suggested that these arise out of a need to exert some kind of independence and autonomy

– even in the face of ongoing dementia. He also proposed an opposite set of approaches that enhance and support the sense of individuality and self – again these are carer characteristics and include: recognition; negotiation; play; relaxation; validation; and facilitation. He asked that carers accept and acknowledge creative actions initiated by the person with dementia, and that caregivers be humble enough to accept whatever gift of kindness or support a person with dementia is able to bestow. For Kitwood, the ideas of being a benefactor or dispenser of charity has no place (Kitwood 1997).

Brooker (2008), working within the Bradford Dementia Group at the University of Bradford, describes what she calls a contemporary approach to person-centred care. When she was first asked to write about person-centred care in 2004 she realised that there was no single definition of what person-centred care really was, although it was mentioned in many policy and care-related documents. Person-centred care was mentioned in terms of individualised care or even a moral imperative.

Since Kitwood's death in 1998, there has been much research into various aspects of care for people with dementia as well as a number of books written by those with dementia discussing the realities of the condition from their perspective – something that was quite rare prior to his death. Brooker (2004) proposed that in keeping with the Kitwood philosophy of person-centred care there are four major aspects or elements – all of these must be present to achieve the goal of effective dementia care. These are:

- valuing people with dementia and those who care for them

- treating people as individuals

- looking at the world from the perspective of the person with dementia

- a positive social environment in which the person with dementia can experience well-being.

VALUING PEOPLE WITH DEMENTIA AND THEIR CARERS

This concerns promoting citizenship, rights and entitlements regardless of cognitive impairment, age or dependency needs. In our society, which tends to stigmatise mental health issues and have ageist attitudes towards older people, workers caring for older people, especially those with dementia, have some of the lowest pay and least respect of all workers in health care. The nurse in paediatric care has a far higher regard than the one in aged care. The parent who cares for her child at home has much more support than a person giving up paid work to care for an elderly relative.

TREATING PEOPLE AS INDIVIDUALS

We should appreciate that all people have a unique history and personality, and physical/mental health, social and economic resources, and that these will affect their response to ageing and dependency and their journey into dementia. In many definitions of person-centred care this has become the major part of the definition. However, for Kitwood and Brooker, this was just one aspect of care. This part of the definition encompasses all the strengths and weaknesses that we see in older people and considers the dementia as part of the overall picture, not the defining part of their identity.

LOOKING AT THE WORLD FROM THE PERSPECTIVE OF THE PERSON WITH DEMENTIA

We should recognise that each person's experience has its own psychological validity and that people act from this perspective, and that empathy with this perspective has its own therapeutic potential. Kitwood (1997) had some suggestions of how this might occur in practice. These include: listening to and reading direct accounts of the experience of living with dementia; using imagination to understand the world of those with dementia; and observing carefully the actions and words of those with dementia (cited in Brooker 2008). The work of Killick and Allen (2001; cited in Brooker 2004) has also been very influential, especially in the UK, to help to examine the world from the perspective of the one with dementia.

A POSITIVE SOCIAL ENVIRONMENT

This is about recognising that all human life is grounded in relationships. Those with dementia need a rich social environment that meets the need for human contact and social growth (Brooker 2004, 2008). Person-centred care takes place within the context of relationships. As the ability to speak is lost then other channels of communication need to be established – there is a need for warm, accepting human contact.

Person-centred care is far more than just treating a person as an individual; Kitwood (1997) proposed person-centred care as a complete package – one that called for societal change as well as change within a care milieu. It has become an ethic of care.

Dementia care mapping

Dementia care mapping (DCM) and person-centred care were both established and described by Kitwood (1997) as a way of ensuring that care was wholly centred on the needs of the person with dementia. I have already described the concepts of person-centred care. Here I will examine how DCM helps to reinforce person-centred care. Kitwood proposed that DCM was a serious and formal way of seeing the world through the lens of the one with dementia.

DCM is a process of observation of the person with dementia over a period of time during the day. After each five-minute time frame, codes are used to record what has happened to that person and the types of behaviour observed during that period. Behaviours are categorised and scored according to the capacity to improve well-being. Interactions are also observed to identify those that provide positive interactions or personal detractors. Kitwood believed that quality of care and well-being for those with dementia is based firmly on the relationships they have around them (Brooker 2005). In order to provide high-quality observations in DCM the observer has to undergo a period of expert training to develop these specialist skills. This can mean that DCM becomes expensive to implement. Using the data gathered from these observations, person-centred care can be implemented that truly reflects the needs of the person with dementia.

In an Australian study (Chenoweth *et al.* 2009) DCM and person-centred care was compared with usual care. They found that although there was no increase in measured quality of care or medication use, agitation was significantly reduced in the groups using DCM and person-centred care. Because agitation causes distress to staff, relatives and the person with dementia, reduction in agitation assisted all members of the care team. They also found that although management were very supportive of the project, it was sometimes difficult to get all staff on side providing consistent care. This is something we have also found when implementing spiritual reminiscence – for many of these activities to have a consistent impact, everyone needs to be committed to the concept. DCM can, however, provide a shared language and assist staff across all aspects of care to have a common goal and can be used as both an evaluative tool as well as a mode of practice development (Brooker 2005).

Art therapy

Art therapy is another way of engaging with those with dementia in a creative and active way through appreciation, observation and actively painting and drawing. There have been a number of studies that have highlighted the benefits of art and art appreciation (MacPherson *et al.* 2009; Rusted, Sheppard and Waller 2006). Hannemann (2006) has found that the expression of creativity 'reinforces essential connections between brain cells, including those responsible for memory', encourages emotional resilience and promotes positive outlook and well-being (p.61). Creative activities, like those engaged in art therapy, may also decrease experiences of isolation and depression (Hannemann 2006).

Music therapy

The role of music in a person's life is not just one of hobby or enjoyment, but the connection to music may occur on a deeper level. Music therapy has been used with dementia patients to decrease agitation and improve memory (Sorrell and Sorrell 2008). It has been found to promote 'positive effects in mood and socialization of patients diagnosed with dementia' (Wall and Duffy 2010, p.112). Music can help to connect a person with dementia with specific emotions and memories in a way that does not require expressive language (Johnson and Johnson 2007). Other studies have demonstrated that music can reduce anxiety (Sung, Chang and Lee 2010) and depression (Chan *et al.* 2009).

Spiritual approaches to care
Pastoral care

Pastoral care of a person with dementia involves exploring an individual's sense of ultimate meaning and acknowledging the individual's core of existence. Provision of pastoral care considers the spiritual development of the individual and is tailored to assist that person in their individual needs (MacKinlay 2002). Usually pastoral care has been delivered on a one-on-one basis, seeing this as a very personal activity and process. Baker (2000) found that intentional pastoral care, nurturing the spiritual dimension, may reduce the prevalence and degree of depression.

Prayer and meditation

The role of prayer in the lives of people with dementia is, like those without dementia, a way of seeking comfort and connection. For those with dementia and difficulty communicating, the symbol and ritual of prayer becomes increasingly important. These rituals can connect individuals with their memories and their experiences of the divine (Hide 2002). In a study of older Americans, Dunn and Horgas (2000) found that the majority (84%) used prayer as a coping mechanism. Marston (2001) argues that residents of nursing homes who are frail and physically limited in their movement and activity may use prayer as a private activity through which they may find meaning in their lives.

The practice of meditation takes many forms, including Zen meditation, transcendental meditation and Christian meditation. Many of these have their origins in Eastern religions and cultures, while Christian meditation, such as contemplative prayer and centring prayer, is grounded within Christian influences (Ferguson, Willemson and Castañeto 2010). Studies have found that meditation practices may have both psychological and physiological benefits (Lindberg 2005; Seeman, Dubin and Seeman 2003). Benefits of meditation for individuals with dementia include decreased agitation, increased relaxation, and reduction in anxiety and depression (Lindberg 2005).

Summary

Dementia is a many-faceted condition that is a collection of signs and symptoms rather than just one disease. The stigma associated with dementia has a considerable impact on both society's approach to those with dementia and on the person's view of themselves. It is important not to lose sight of the person in dementia and to maintain that sense of identity and individuality. Kitwood's work and the continuation of this by other researchers highlights how people with dementia are marginalised in our community and are frequently consigned to the 'living dead'. However, while there may not yet be a cure for dementia, there are a number of approaches to care that can enhance the lives of those with dementia – and in some cases reduce or slow the amount of memory loss.

3

Investigating Spiritual Reminiscence

The experience of working closely with one person, Christine Bryden (Boden), over a number of years from her diagnosis with early-onset dementia proved to be an exciting and challenging time for Elizabeth (MacKinlay 2011). It was now time to test what had been learnt within this continuing journey with Christine. That had been an in-depth study of one person, and now it was time to ask if a similar process of spiritual reminiscence could be used effectively with other people who have dementia. The direction for our initial study came from questions from Christine as she faced this diagnosis; how could she find meaning in what she was experiencing? At that time, Christine was engaged in small groups of people who had dementia, run by Alzheimer's Australia local branches.

We obtained our first grant, from the University of Canberra to conduct small groups over a six-week or five-month period; the study was titled 'The search for meaning: Quality of life for the person with dementia'. Funding only allowed for a one-year pilot programme. In total 22 people took part in this initial project. Findings from the pilot project identified the importance of relationship for people with dementia, but did not provide sufficient knowledge on working with participants for the development of programmes that might be used with people who have dementia. Comparison with a previous study found the need for intimacy does not seem to diminish in later life (MacKinlay 2001a); in this study this was apparently also the case for the person with dementia. However, when dementia is part of the scene it complicates relationship patterns.

In the pilot study the admission point to an aged care facility was identified as an important transition time, when these people with dementia may be particularly at risk of isolation. It recommended strategies be developed to assist new residents to develop relationships with others in the care setting, both staff and residents. The pilot study also identified the need of staff in aged care facilities to learn skills of facilitating small group work for people with dementia.

The final report of the pilot study noted that physical care is not enough and contended that some so-called disruptive behaviours may be reduced when people with dementia *feel* cared for. Finally, the pilot study affirmed that further work was needed to develop effective ways of connecting with these people.

The objectives of the second study were to:

- examine how people experience dementia
- explore how meaning and quality of life can be achieved by and for people who have dementia
- explore the concept of personhood and respect for persons with dementia
- develop effective strategies to improve quality of life for those with dementia
- help families and staff to find meaningful ways to interact with persons who are experiencing communication difficulties in dementia.

The use of spiritual reminiscence was examined in depth and is the main focus of this book. This study was made possible with the award of an Australian Research Council (ARC) Linkage Grant (2002–2005): 'Finding meaning in the experience of dementia: The place of spiritual reminiscence work'.

In summary, then, we have conducted five years of study into assisting people with dementia to find meaning in their experiences. Much of this work has been directed towards refining the process of facilitating spiritual reminiscence for use with people with dementia. This project addresses both an important area for study and a difficult one methodologically. However, the researchers believe that this is an important area to develop. The study was a collaborative project between Anglican Retirement Community Services, Diocese of Canberra and Goulburn, Wesley Gardens UnitingCare Ageing and Mirinjani Retirement Services. Residential facilities were located in Canberra (three facilities), Merimbula (two facilities) and Sydney (two facilities).

Methodology

As little research had been done in this area, it was important not to foreclose on any important avenues of concern; thus a mixed-method approach was chosen for the study. First, the conceptual framework for the study was qualitative, using grounded theory (Glaser and Strauss 1967; Morse 1992). In-depth interviewing (Minichiello *et al.* 1995) was used to tap into the experience of dementia for the participants. This methodology is the most appropriate as it allows the individual freedom to express themselves, and so is valuable in a new research area such as spirituality, dementia and ageing. Methods of recording data also took account of non-verbal communications by observation of participants during the sessions, for those who have language difficulties in moderate to severe dementia. This helped build an understanding of the participants' experiences of dementia, communication styles and difficulties, and thus increase the understanding of the condition for carers and relatives. The study design had originally allowed for relatives to be used to fill in the details of a life review for individuals who had moderate communication difficulties, but in the process of the study, this was not found necessary. In Gibson's (1994) experience with severely demented people, a number of them were able to give a detailed life history themselves. However, because the process used in this study focused on group interactions, potential participants who had little remaining language were not included in the groups.

The qualitative methods chosen examined meaning for the individual by the process of, first, in-depth interview and, second, spiritual reminiscence. The questions allowed exploration of the search for meaning and hope in these people and the strategies they use in finding meaning in their experience of dementia. Meanings ascribed by participants to past life experiences were explored, seeking to find meaning in the light of dementia, in the process of the weekly sessions of spiritual reminiscence. Third, a research assistant observed and recorded participant communications, both verbal and non-verbal, emotional responses, and strategies used by individuals during group sessions, relating to quality and meaning of life. This study examined how dementia is experienced by the individual, taking account of both their individual life story and then their engagement in the small group process.

Quantitative measures were also included in the study to gauge the effectiveness of the spiritual reminiscence work. Data were collected for demographics and measures of cognitive status using the Mini Mental State Examination (MMSE: Folstein, Folstein and McHugh 1975) and a behaviour rating scale (INTERACT: Baker and Dowling 1995).

Measure of behaviour related to weekly group sessions

A before–after behaviour rating scale (INTERACT: Baker and Dowling 1995) was used to measure changes in behaviour from before to after the group sessions. This form has been tested for reliability and validity and used in a number of studies (e.g. Baker *et al.* 2001).

The main themes of the form assessed for mood, speech, relating to others, relating to the environment, need for prompting and stimulation level. Twelve behaviours are charted from observation within ten minutes before and during the ten minutes after the group on a Likert scale of not at all to nearly all the time (1–5). The INTERACT questions are in Table 3.1.

The qualitative methods

A qualitative method was employed, with grounded theory being employed to identify themes in the qualitative data. Several reasons made the use of grounded theory most appropriate for this study. First, it was a little-studied area, and the use of grounded theory is valuable in examining participant concerns and interests, building data into themes and collecting data to a point at which no new themes emerge (saturation of data) (Glaser and Strauss 1967; Morse 1992; Morse and Field 1995; Strauss and Corbin 1990). In this inductive process the participants are crucial, as it is their words that form the basis of the study shaping the outcomes through the data that is collected, rather than having a structure imposed on them externally through a questionnaire (MacKinlay 2006).

Judging credibility

Based on Glaser and Strauss (1967, 1999) it can be seen that the multiple comparisons used in this study of the weekly collection of data through the process of small groups add to the credibility of the data obtained.

Multiple comparison groups make the credibility of the theory considerably greater. By precisely detailing the many similarities and differences of the various comparison groups, the analyst knows, better than if only one or a few social systems had been studied, under what sets of structural conditions the hypotheses are minimised and maximised, and hence to what kinds of social structures the theory is applicable (Glaser and Strauss 1967, 1999).

Ethics approval

The University of Canberra Ethics Committee granted ethics approval in March 2002. Subsequently, when the project transferred to Charles Sturt University, ethics approval was obtained in 2003. Ethics approval was obtained from all participating residential aged care facilities. Once consent had been gained from each participant and their relative, an in-depth interview was completed by one of the principal researchers, prior to the collection of demographics and initial data of cognitive status.

Table 3.1 The INTERACT questions, as designed by Baker and Dowling (1995)	
Mood 1. Tearful/sad 2. Happy/content 3. Fearful/anxious 4. Confused	**Speech** 5. Talked spontaneously
Relating to others 6. Related well to other staff/patients	**Relating to the environment** 7. Attentive/responding to/focused on environment
Need for prompting 8. Did things from own initiative	**Stimulation level** 9. Wandering, restless or aggressive *(undesirably active)* 10. Enjoying self, active or alert *(desirably active)* 11. Bored, inactive or sleeping inappropriately *(undesirably inactive)* 12. Relaxed, content or sleeping appropriately *(desirably inactive)*

Participant recruitment

Letters of information and invitation to participate in the study were given to potential participants and relatives of residents with a medical diagnosis of dementia, who could speak and understand English, and were able to mobilise adequately to join a small discussion group. Researchers gave information sessions in the different aged care facilities, to both residents and families. (Staff also attended information sessions.)

Consent to participate in the research was on the basis that signatures of both the person with dementia and their legal guardian or next of kin would be obtained. Where one or the other refused to give consent, then we would not include that person in our study. We did this to protect the prospective participants, and to honour both them and their family member or legal guardian. In all instances, we, as researchers, did not approach potential participants for the study. Instead, we met with staff and explained the study, gave them the letters of information and the consent forms, and asked them to approach residents with the invitation to participate in the study. It was obviously not appropriate for anyone from the research team to invite participation as we could have been seen to place these already vulnerable people under pressure to be part of the study, to gain more participants for the study.

Staff recruiting and training

Staff positions were advertised and recruited for each residential aged care facility. Training sessions were held for all staff working on the project, at the centres where they were employed. Group sessions were facilitated by either diversional therapists or pastoral carers. The study design nominated diversional therapists as the group facilitators. However, in a couple of situations, one arising from an accident that happened to the designated diversional therapist just before the group was due to begin, it was necessary to find a replacement quickly. A pastoral carer who was already working in this section of the aged care facility was the obvious choice, because she was available, she had very good group skills and knew the residents. In both situations where a pastoral carer was used, the group outcomes were very good, with participants expressing satisfaction and enjoyment of the groups.

Sample

The sample consisted of 113 people aged 62–96 who had been diagnosed with dementia, were able to speak and understand English and were in institutional care. The MMSE served as a basis of inclusion. The sample was invited from onsite at each of the facilities of Anglican Retirement Community Services (Canberra and Merimbula), Mirinjani Retirement Village in Canberra and Wesley Gardens Aged Care in Sydney. It was not possible to include a group of those living in the community who were receiving Community Aged Care Packages (CACPs) and serviced from these aged care facilities. (CACPs are a means of providing a range of care services for older people delivered in their own homes, as an alternative to care in an aged care facility.) The main problem was lack of staff and, in one case, a perceived need by the staff to concentrate on physical activities when these people came to the facility, together with, in one instance, suspicion of a programme that included spirituality.

ASSIGNMENT TO GROUPS

The plan was to have 22 treatment groups and two control groups, consisting of two group types, short (six weeks) and long term (24 weeks). In the final study, 27 groups were included (this allowed for the lack of individual cases being followed). A total of 113 people participated in the 27 discussion groups (of three to six people), which were conducted over the period September 2003 to December 2004. Smaller group sizes were used for participants who had more compromised verbal abilities.

The inclusion of short- and long-term groups is based on the work of Yale (1995), who had established six-week therapeutic groups. Her group work was adopted at a number of settings in Australia as well as the USA; however, from our experience of working with people who have dementia, it seemed that six weeks might not be sufficient time for people with dementia to benefit, and that longer group support might be more effective, but there was no work that had tested this.

This study aimed to study differences in the responses of participants over the shorter and longer groups. There were six 24-week groups, each group consisting of three to five people (smaller numbers where participants were more cognitively compromised). One group was from a rural aged care facility, while the other five groups were drawn from urban facilities.

The short-term cohort consisted of 18 groups: four groups from dementia-specific units (including one group from a rural setting), with the remaining groups from a mixture of aged care facilities. One group was composed of a single ethnic group.

The details of the small groups are summarised in Table 3.2.

Table 3.2 Location, duration and completion of small groups			
LOCATION	6-WEEK GROUPS completed	24-WEEK GROUPS completed	INCOMPLETE GROUPS
Urban (site 1)	4	2	1
Rural (site 1)	2	1	1
Urban (site 2)	2		
Rural (site 2)	2		
Urban (site3)	2	2	
Urban (site 4)	4		
Urban (site 5)	2	1	1
TOTAL	18	6	3

Staff focus groups

In addition to the data collection of the small groups, which obviously involved the people with dementia, it was thought important to gain some understanding of staff perceptions of the spiritual reminiscence. Staff caring for the study participants were invited to take part in focus groups after the end of the project. They had the opportunity to share what they had found by being involved in the care of these people during the project. They were also asked for their perceptions of changes to resident behaviour, and staff morale would be measured.

Data collection

Demographic data, in-depth interviews and evaluation of cognitive function (using MMSE) and spiritual/meaning in life assessments were done prior to participation. The Bird Memory Scale and MMSE were administered again at three months, six months and then six months after completion of the interventions, for most groups. However, there was some difficulty in following up with participants after the completion of the groups, due to a number of factors, including staff changes, participants being moved to other facilities, and deaths of a few participants. Each in-depth interview was recorded, transcribed and analysed for themes. These interviews provided valuable data to build on the study already completed in this area with cognitively intact elderly people (MacKinlay 1998, 2001a, 2001b). Groups were held once a week during the study period. A style of within-group control was used, having the assessments done weekly, including the INTERACT behaviour scale, but no treatments for four weeks before beginning the group sessions. One further group did not follow the set questions on meaning that were set out and taught in the training programme. This group showed no significant interaction, so in effect served as a control group as the programme was not run as designed for this group. It had been planned to work with 15 people on a one-to-one basis, but facility staffing did not allow for this higher level of input.

The longer group process: challenges for the research process

In practice, the running of the longer groups, over 24 weeks, proved challenging for the research process. Factors included staff constraints, lack of extra funding, the vulnerability of the participants and lack of respect that was needed for them in a research process. With the best intentions of staff and participants, it could not be guaranteed that participants would be present. Illness, other appointments, increasing frailty and, in a few cases, death of a group member intervened, thus lowering the attendance rates. While attendance rates were good, missing data could not be avoided in this real-world situation.

Results

Quantitative measures analysed by SPSS were: demographic data; MMSE, with mean of 18.12 at entry and 16.09 at exit (only four groups at final test); and a behavioural rating scale, INTERACT, used before and after every session of every group.

Demographics

Of the 113 participants, there were 98 women (87%) and 15 men (13%). Other demographic information is missing for seven of these women and one of the men. The mean age of the remaining 105 participants was 83.37 years (s.d. 7.20); for 14 of the men it was 82.1 years (s.d. 9.9, range 53–93 years) and for 91 of the women it was 83.6 years (s.d. 6.7, range 62–97 years). Three people (two women; one man) were interviewed and tested for inclusion in the programme but did not choose to participate.

Information about education was often not recorded by residential facilities, and hard to obtain. This was true of nearly one quarter of the sample. Table 3.3 provids a list of the education levels attained by the participants.

Most people in this study were Australian born (77 or 68.1%), although none were of ATSI (Aboriginal and Torres Strait Islander) origin; 12 came from the UK (10.6%), another 12 from Europe (10.6%), one from South Africa and two from Sri Lanka (2.7% outside Europe). There was no information recorded for nine participants (8.0%). One hundred and two (90.3%) people were living in hostels for the aged at the time of the study, ten in nursing homes (8.8%), and one was supported by an aged care package.

Table 3.3 Education levels attained by participants		
LEVEL REACHED	**NUMBER**	**% OF 113** **(all participants)**
No schooling	1	0.9
Completed primary	8	7.1
Part high school	22	19.5
Completed high school	16	14.2
Trade training	14	12.4
Diploma/degree	12	10.6
Postgraduate	6	5.3
Unknown	26	23.0
Missing	8	7.1

Cognitive function before and after the programme

Cognitive function was estimated by using Folstein's MMSE. Most people were assessed before commencing the programme. Some groups had follow-up tests after the end of the course. Some initial test results are missing.

All participants had to have a diagnosis of dementia to be accepted into the study. It is noted that, although the normal cut-off point for dementia is 24 and below out of a possible score of 30, there are known cases of people with a diagnosis of dementia who have scores of 30/30. It is considered to be rare (Shiroky *et al.* 2007). Several participants in this study had an MMSE score of 30/30; they had a diagnosis of dementia, and we made the decision to keep them in the study.

The cognitive test results can be found in Tables 3.4 and 3.5.

Table 3.4 Cognitive test results – initial testing of all participants			
TEST	GROUP (n)	MEAN SCORE (s.d.)	MEDIAN SCORE (range)
MMSE – initial test	Whole group (93)	18.12 (7.65)	19.00 (0–30)
	Men (15)	19.73 (7.03)	20.00 (4–30)
	Women (78)	17.81 (7.77)	18.25 (0–30)

Table 3.5 Cognitive test results – final testing (four groups only)			
TEST	GROUP (n)	MEAN SCORE (s.d.)	MEDIAN SCORE (range)
MMSE – final test	Whole group (22)	16.09 (7.16)	16.50 (4–30)
	Men (1)	18.00 (individual)	one score only
	Women (21)	16.00 (7.33)	16.00 (4–30)

Data analysis

Demographic data were analysed using SPSS. The other quantitative data were analysed using SPSS, with MANOVA used for checking multivariate relationships between group members and the group over time. The qualitative statistical computer package QSR N6 was chosen because of the large quantities of data to be analysed. The in-depth interviews and weekly group transcripts were analysed using N6. Subsequently, data has been re-analysed using NVivo8 to gain from recent advances in the rigour of the qualitative analysis programme.

INTERACT scale analysis

Analysis of the data from the INTERACT scale proved complex. Factor analysis was performed on the scale, with items grouped as used by Baker and Dowling (1995). Factor analysis failed to support their assumptions on the assigned factors, and the data was re-examined to find factors and the items from the data that accounted for these factors.[1]

Factor analysis produced three new factors: Connecting, Fearful/agitated/despair and Self-transcendence/integrity. The items associated with each of the factors are set out in Table 3.6.

Table 3.6 Results of factor analysis[2]	
Factor	**Item associated with factor**
Factor 1: Connecting	10. Enjoying self, active or alert *(desirably active)* 7. Attentive/responding to/focused on environment 6. Related well to other staff/patients 2. Happy/content
Factor 2: Fearful/agitated/despair	9. Wandering, restless or aggressive *(undesirably active)* 1. Tearful/sad 3. Fearful/anxious 4. Confused
Factor 3: Self-transcendence/integrity	5. Talked spontaneously 8. Did things from own initiative 11. Bored, inactive or sleeping inappropriately *(undesirably inactive)* 12. Relaxed, content or sleeping appropriately *(desirably inactive)*

It is noted that item 12, relaxed, content or sleeping appropriately, was removed from the items on the basis of reliability estimates with it present versus absent. The removal of this item from Factor 3 results in reliability statistics as follows – Factor 1: Connecting, Cronbach's Alpha .871 (four items); Factor 2: Fearful/agitated/despair, Cronbach's Alpha .819 (four items); and Factor 3: Self-transcendence/integrity, Cronbach's Alpha .748 (three items). All new factors have acceptable reliability levels.

PRE-SESSION VERSUS POST-SESSION SCORES

The INTERACT scale was recorded before and after each weekly session; however, it is more likely that effects would be seen over the longer term, unless changes occurred in the group session time.

1 We are grateful to Professor Michael Kiernan for his assistance with statistical analysis.

2 Item order is according to the strength of association of the item with the factor.

It is noted that the majority of groups were the shorter groups of six weeks' duration. Detecting statistically significant changes in the longer groups lacked sufficient statistical power to be of real value, due to the small number of 24-week groups. The further analysis of the first six-week session across all groups, short and long, is reported in further detail below.

Detailed analysis assumed that the six sessions represented six different interventions, and each session had a different main theme (see Table 3.7). It could be assumed that as these six themes were repeated through the longer groups, in the same sequence, that the first block of six sessions would be the best evaluation of any changes in participant responses to the different themes as this would be a purer assessment of the individual contribution of the intervention, as it was the first time this process was experienced by the participants.

Testing all the groups together has more statistical power to detect any effects since all participants of all the groups were included. However, a note of caution is raised here, in that people with dementia may take longer to take in what is happening in the process, and may not show changes until they have been engaged in the group process for a longer period of time than would be the case with cognitively competent older adults. Thus the short groups lasting only six weeks may not be a good guide to the performance of these people in the longer time frame.

Table 3.7 The main weekly themes	
Week	**Main theme**
Week 1	Life-meaning
Week 2	Relationships, isolation and connecting
Week 3	Hopes, fears and worries
Week 4	Growing older and transcendence
Week 5	Spiritual and religious beliefs
Week 6	Spiritual and religious practices

It was not possible to tell from the quantitative data whether there were differences between responses of participants to the different topics. However, it was possible to examine the three factors across the six sessions. The best outcomes were obtained for Factor 1: Connecting, with significant moves between pre- and post-sessions at Session 1: significant at (two-tailed) .024; Session 3: significant at .001; Session 4: significant at .001; Session 5: .016; and Session 6: .002. Factor 2: Fearful/agitated/despair only showed significance at Session 4: .020. No significance was found in Factor 3 over the first six weeks.

To determine if any changes occurred over the longer term, comparison was made between the corresponding session in the first six-week session and in the last session of the 24-week groups. In this, for Factor 1: Connecting, significant changes of .001 in Session 2 were found; in Session 4, .026; while in Session 5 it was significant at .000. There were no significant changes for Factor 2: Fearful/agitated/despair. There was one significant change for Factor 3: Self-transcendence/integrity in Session 5 (compared with Session 23) at .009.

It was possible to see in the qualitative data that participants responded better to some topics than others. Part of the differences could be associated with the facilitator style of communication and ease with leading discussion on the different topics. For instance, some facilitators were not comfortable with sharing discussion about faith, or religion, even though they themselves attended church. Group members seemed to respond readily to the comfort levels of the facilitator, either responding more, or having less to say. Participant input also varied according to their individual areas of concern and interest.

Comments on analysis

From the in-depth interviews of spiritual reminiscence conducted prior to assignment to a group, analysis of themes of life-meaning showed that, in these people with dementia, meaning was almost synonymous with relationship, or connecting with others. This is actually borne out by the statistical results. Regardless of the fact that we often say that people with moderate or more severe dementia do not recognise people, connecting with others is vital to them. This was clearly backed in the data obtained in the weekly transcripts of the group sessions.

What did we discover in the longer groups? It is noted that Factor 3: Self-transcendence/integrity, in Session 5 (compared with Session 23) at .009, showed that for the measures of talked spontaneously, did things from own initiative and bored, inactive or sleeping inappropriately, all of which can be seen as signs of self-transcendence, there were significant changes over the duration of the longer groups.

NVivo8 showed that interactions within groups increased. There was increased connecting between group members that was not initiated by the facilitator, and there were signs of friendships developing. It was apparent from the weekly research assistant journal and increasing interactions observed within the sessions in the longer term, and seen in the qualitative analysis, that the groups were of even more benefit in the longer term.

The qualitative analysis

Qualitative data were collected through audio-taping and transcribing in-depth interviews of all participants and all weekly group sessions. A research assistant also observed all group sessions and maintained a journal of non-verbal interactions. Qualitative data were analysed using QSR N6 (later re-analysed with NVivo8 as this new package became available) and grounded theory.

From our studies into spiritual reminiscence we have seen that communication strategies aimed at allowing the person with dementia time to consider answers in a small supportive group can greatly enhance their ability to talk of meaningful issues. In small groups, discussing issues of spiritual reminiscence, we often observe thoughtful answers and considerable insight into their situation. The ability of the person to respond, however, is frequently linked to the quality of the facilitator of the group. Listening to transcripts, we can hear instances of not allowing the person time to respond, putting words into the person's mouth or answering for them. Some of these communication styles match with Kitwood's (1997) claim of 'malignant social psychology'.

We often observed in transcripts thoughtful answers and considerable insight into their situation. The ability of the person to respond was frequently linked to the attitudes and communication style of the group facilitator. Within sessions, participants also supported each other through touch and empathetic expression.

Even asking 'difficult' questions has elicited many responses. When we ask about meaning in life, most people talk about their family – their parents, siblings or children. They make excuses for why their children do not visit regularly. Although they seemed to lack a sense of time for other activities, they would get themselves ready for the group sessions without prompting, and on the right day and time.

Following the groups, some of the participants have been noted to be animatedly chatting as they go to the dining room. Research assistant journals recorded instances of participants spontaneously speaking to each other outside the group, making new friends. Once separated from the reminiscence group they attempt to engage the people on each side of them at dinner, but soon give up as they receive no response. Again, they become listless, quiet and uninterested in what is going on around them. What is it about the spiritual reminiscence group that encourages this interaction? At the conclusion of one group meeting, one participant said, 'Thank you for this. We do not get to talk about these things usually.'

The themes from the in-depth interviews (of the 113 participants) are shown in Table 3.8.

Table 3.8 Analysis of the in-depth interviews for the whole project: Themes	

1. Ultimate meaning
  a. Meaning
  b. Image of God
  c. Joy
  d. Good things in life
	2. Response to meaning
	  a. Being sad
	  b. Church attendance
	  c. Meditation and spiritual practices
	  d. Praying
	  e. Faith
	  f. Negative associations with religion

3. Relationships and connectedness
  a. Relationships
  b. Grief
  c. Spiritual and emotional supports
  d. Feeling lonely
  e. Regrets and guilt
  f. Living in residential aged care
	4. Vulnerability and transcendence
	  a. Worries
	  b. Hardest things
	  c. Fears
	  d. Communication patterns and difficulties
	    i. Being lost for words
	  e. Awareness of cognitive disabilities
	  f. Perceptions of health
	    i. Health and disabilities
	  g. Living with dementia
	  h. Resilience

5. Wisdom and final meanings
  a. Memories in general
  b. Growing older
  c. Coping skills
  d. Dying process and attitudes towards death
  e. Activities in the aged care residence
  f. Vocation
  g. Insight
	6. Hope versus despair
	  a. Hope
	  b. Despair

Participants found greatest meaning in life through family and relationships. Saddest events in their lives were the loss of parents that occurred when they were children. The majority of participants had a faith in God and had been active participants in their church. In many cases this continued into their life at the aged care facility. They expressed the hope that they would keep their health, and the majority had no fears. All were ready to accept death when it came and felt they had enjoyed a good life. This contrasted with findings from a previous study of independent-living older and cognitively intact people, where 100 per cent of participants held fears for their future well-being.

There is abundant, rich material from the many individual and group sessions and this is presented in the chapters where it is of most relevance. The richness of the data was almost overwhelming, and we look forward to sharing this with you in the subsequent chapters.

Summary

This chapter has outlined the rationale for the study on which this book is based. It has demonstrated the need for such work and the methods used to study older people with dementia and where they find meaning in the experience of dementia.

Results of analysis have been outlined to help the reader to see what lies behind the process of examining spiritual reminiscence with this group of vulnerable people.

PART 2

Listening to Those with Dementia: The Findings

4

Autonomy and the Older Person with Dementia

Ethically, the first question to be asked about the person who has dementia is – Who is this person? Stokes (2010) has raised a number of important issues about the person in dementia through his clinical practice. Reflecting on the nature of dementia he asked:

> Could it be that we no longer see them as people whose feelings need to be acknowledged and their opinions valued? Are we seduced by the simplicity and authority of the disease-model that not only fails to talk of people, but also absolves us of all responsibility? Can we really say that whatever a person with dementia does, it is because they have dementia? (p.54)

These are vital questions of a deeply ethical nature. The way we relate to and with people who have dementia, and the way that we provide care, will be influenced by the way we see the person who has dementia. Do we only see the disease model? Do we see the person who has dementia as a whole person? Do we automatically attribute any distressing behaviours to the disease? Sometimes, even the opportunities open to people with dementia are limited by what carers and the person with dementia see as possible. Often this is framed by what the person 'can't do' instead of endeavouring to find what they 'can do'. This chapter includes the discussion of issues that we discovered during the process of this research, informed by the very vulnerability of these people. So, while it is a chapter on ethics applied to dementia issues in general, it is importantly illustrated with material from the research project.

The chapter engages with issues of identity in dementia, and ethical behaviour of the person with dementia and their care providers, on the basis of loss of cognition. Ethical issues cover a range of topics, from truth telling, including being told of their diagnosis of dementia, to capacity to give consent for health care, to end-of-life issues. Autonomy is an important aspect of these ethical issues. To a large extent, what is understood about the nature of the person with dementia drives the agenda for the shape of ethical behaviour towards people who have dementia, and to an extent also what is possible for the person themselves.

How do we see the person who has dementia?

- Is it as one who has lost their voice?
- One who cannot make decisions?
- One who cannot take responsibility for themselves and their health care and well-being?
- One who is now dependent and must be protected from risk?
- Or as a partner in care?
- One who has communication and memory challenges?
- Still a real person with hopes and dreams, with possibilities open to the future?

Often, when a person has a diagnosis of dementia, conversations begin to bypass them, and healthcare providers speak with family members rather than the person with dementia, even when the person with dementia is in the same room. This is a very clear indication that the person who has the diagnosis of dementia is no longer really regarded as a person. Malcolm Goldsmith was one of the first to ask the questions of people *with* dementia, rather than those who care for them, in his book *Hearing the Voice of People with Dementia* (1996).

The worth and dignity of the person

The non-negotiable value and worth of the human person is recognised in the Abrahamic faiths, acknowledging that human beings are made in the image of God. In humanistic terms too, the value of the human person is recognised as being irreducible (Gastmans and De Lepeleire 2010). In this context, the right of the individual person to live their life as an independent autonomous being, who can make decisions without regard for any other person or persons, is affirmed. In this understanding of the person, the worth and dignity of the person is constant, regardless of cognitive capacity or any other consideration. Murphy (2006) notes that the concept of person precedes that of mental life. This is an important consideration of what it means to be a person. It is not the body only, nor the mental capacities alone, that make a person, but a combination comprising the whole person.

Not only is the person of value, but the person-in-relationship is recognised as being of importance, and this is also acknowledged in dementia:

> Persons with dementia are situated, among other things, within a familial, cultural, and historical context. The growth of demented persons is to a large extent based on a balance between autonomy and solidarity, not just on individual self-determination. (Gastmans and De Lepeleire 2010, p.82)

Thus issues of autonomy are seen in a different light and wider context of community and relationship. One term that describes this newer way of understanding the concept of autonomy is relational autonomy, meaning that we can only be understood in relationship with others. This is a crucial concept for understanding and affirming the identity of the person who has dementia.

Ethics, spirituality and dementia

The context in which dementia is approached will largely determine the ethical perspective in which the person with dementia and their family is seen. The view of ethics from a biomedical perspective will emphasise cognitive status and loss, disabilities and the diminished status and responsibilities of the person. It may mean that the person is seen only as a disease that needs to be treated, and as dementia is not generally regarded as being able to be cured, then there is little value placed on the medical care of these people. A view seen from a social perspective may these days allow for a much more positive outlook and ethical approach, affirming the personhood of the one with dementia, and seeing them as of value even while losing much of their cognitive functions. Much has been done in recent decades, particularly through the work of Tom Kitwood (1997), to change attitudes towards and about people with dementia.

The view from a pastoral or theological perspective acknowledges the person with dementia as being made in the image of God and, consequently, issues of love, justice and mercy override the issues of the medical diagnosis. Perhaps topics of ethics, spirituality and dementia are a volatile mix. On the one hand, it is important when working with people who have cognitive disabilities to recognise their disability produces vulnerability. However, often we address issues of vulnerability in people with dementia by overprotecting them and removing from them all responsibility and need for engagement with others. On the other hand, we may need to learn how to enable these people to live more effectively in the midst of their disabilities. A balance is needed between what the person can still do and what they can't do. This will change from day to day and person to person. It is all too easy to make one rule fit all. At all times, the value of the person is affirmed, regardless of their vulnerability and disability.

The problems with autonomy in dementia

Autonomy has been clearly identified during the 20th century as possibly the single most important ethical principle in biomedical ethics. Liberal Western societies have placed high value on human autonomy. This has gone hand in hand with the development of the importance of the individual as the highest value within a society. It is only in recent times that some authors have begun to raise concerns about the possible implications for society and the well-being of humanity where these attitudes prevail, while at the same time the importance of community and relationship has become relatively neglected.

The concept of autonomy views individual rights to be considered without reference to others, unless the individual's rights impinge on others. The difficulty with autonomy as a basis for the highest value within a society is that there are times when a person cannot be autonomous. In fact, in reality, in complex Western societies, real autonomy is a false goal and value. We are all ultimately interdependent human beings. Dementia severely tests the ethical principle of autonomy, based as it is on the cognitive capacity of the individual. The main issues here are issues of competence; a person with dementia does not become incompetent in all areas, and may be quite competent in decision-making one day, but not the next, and competent in some domains, while not in others. Their ability or degree of difficulty in communicating their wishes may complicate the decision-making process even further.

A perceived lack of autonomy for the person with dementia has implications for care and, associated with this, provisions for care, which may include research. Further, care provider understanding of autonomy in the particular person with dementia can be affected by the care provider's understanding of personhood. This will have a direct effect on the *way* care is given, and the choices available to the person. If people with dementia are seen simply to have progressive loss of cognitive function, and that the disease is solely one of biological decline, then it is easy to see that these people, once diagnosed, may simply be provided with basic physical care.

Yet, an ethical stance to this disease sees a number of other factors that are important in the definition of the disease and the sense of hope that patients may hold. Likewise, the hopes and aspirations for care providers will also be dependent on the view of these possibilities. While Kitwood's (1997) work has been crucial in this new way of seeing dementia, nearly two decades after his work these principles are not universally practised in dementia care.

A way that cares – ethically

There have been several ethically focused studies that demonstrate that the way care is delivered can make a difference for the person with dementia. The authors of one early study asserted that it is not just the biomedical view of this disease that has to be taken account of, but the 'complexity of the human experience of dementia' (Sixsmith, Stilwell and Copeland 1993, p.994). Sixsmith *et al.*, in their study conducted in three nursing homes for elderly mentally ill people, used strategies of encouraging independence, individual rights and personal fulfilment. They found changes in behaviour and, specifically, dependency levels over the study period. These changes were particularly marked in the one home measured over a 36-month period, where residents were admitted having 'management problems'. Their dependency levels improved, and they attributed this to 'rementia' or, in other words, recovery of some cognitive abilities (Sixsmith *et al.* 1993). Kitwood (1997) had suggested that a process of rementia may occur in some cases where good social care is provided.

Following similar principles, Moniz-Cook, Stokes and Agar (2003) conducted a study of five cases of psychosocial interventions with people exhibiting difficult behaviour and dementia. They found that individualised interventions of psychosocial care in a person-centred mode were effective in alleviating distress in the people with dementia, and helped staff to understand and deliver appropriate care. In their study outcomes they noted: 'Thus challenging behaviour is not inevitably the symptomatic consequence of neuro-degeneration, but the outcome of psychosocial factors that are responsive not simply to control, but to amelioration and resolution' (Moniz-Cook *et al.* 2003, p.204). This demonstrated that how we see and interact with the person with dementia is important.

Restrictions of freedom and deception

One of the ways that protective strategies are practised in dementia care is to restrict the freedom of people with dementia. It is important to ask: Is it legitimate to restrict the freedoms of people who have dementia? For instance, quite a number of people with dementia wander, and thus may present a danger to themselves and others. But is it appropriate that they should have restrictions on their movements, and if so, what kind of restrictions might be appropriate? It is often thought that residents with dementia do not notice that they are locked in a section of a care facility. Yet, during our small group work, this was a topic of conversation, raised by participants in one of the groups, when a new procedure of security had been put in place.

The dilemma in this case was the responsibility for safety of these residents versus allowing freedom. The following is taken from a discussion in one of the group sessions, with the issue raised by a resident under the broad question from the group facilitator of worries that the participants might have:

Facilitator: Are there any worries about your daily life here, anything here that is a worry?

Rose: Oh well of course they gummed up one of our, our things to go through, so I have got to get some, my grandson tomorrow, I said to him you have got to get permission for us to go through the door.

Facilitator: Oh yes that's right.

Rose: That's the new thing, that's a worry.

Facilitator: Yeah.

Rose: Well that was silly, that was a very silly sort of thing, but they did it.

Facilitator: Yes.

Rose: Six months, six, six weeks ago they did that.

Alice: Well that's because missing at the moment, so many things have been stolen, people running into places, and snatching money or whatever.

Facilitator: And some people are wandering away and getting out onto the main road. Which is a bit of a worry, you know, so that's why it was made secure, so people can't get out.

Rose: Well I just really, I heard it was one man who died, and then they locked up all sorts of things, and it was just a pain in the neck.

Facilitator: Mmm.

Rose: So I can't really commend it.

Facilitator: No, no it's hard for you.

Rose: Well the thing was they were very smart, they did not ask our opinion about it, they just said, we will do it.

Facilitator: Mmm.

Rose: So I really can't commend it. (*laughs*)

In the group meeting a week later, Rose took up the theme again:

Rose: So we both [she and her husband] made, and they said there is a place for you also, and of course then they changed all the rules, which I was not very happy about, and locked the doors and everything.

This excerpt illustrates the complexity of working with these vulnerable people, of their frustrations at having their movements restricted, but at the same time the responsibility of the organisation and staff to provide a safe environment for the residents, especially those with dementia. In the excerpt from the transcript of the group session the facilitator gives the residents the opportunity to talk about issues that are of concern to them; she supports and explains as appropriate. It seems there may have been a breakdown in communication of the proposed changes to security in the building, and it is also possible that the residents did not remember explanations that had been given. What is important in this example is that the facilitator listened to and affirmed the residents in their concerns. This is ethics in practice in residential aged care.

Another issue that could have been raised here is that of deception, which Kitwood (1997) wrote of. It is easy to deceive people who have lost cognitive capacity. This was not apparent in the example above, as the conversation within the group session was open and honest. It is not known how the process of bringing in the new security measures in the building was established.

Interpersonal relationships: 'Behaviours' in dementia

How is behaviour related to ethics? It is central to ethics, as every way that we act or 'behave' has to do with relationship. How we act, or respond to the acts or behaviour of another person, is always ethical (or unethical). We often hear of 'behaviours' in dementia and how these should be managed. As human beings, we all exhibit behaviours as long as we are alive. Perhaps 'behaviour' used in dementia language means difficult or disruptive behaviour. It is worth noting that, in any interaction between people, both parties in the interaction 'behave'. We tend to respond to each other, often in response to what the other person has said or done we impute motives to them for the behaviour that we perceive. And this is important; it is our perception of the behaviour that we so often act upon, and sometimes we could just be wrong. Tom Kitwood's (1997) list of malignant social psychology is a useful one to keep in mind for examining our assessment and response to behaviours of people who have dementia. Kitwood outlined 17 different elements of malignant social psychology sometimes seen in dementia care: treachery, disempowerment, infantilisation, intimidation, labelling, stigmatisation, outpacing, invalidation, banishment, objectification, ignoring, imposition, withholding, accusation, disruption, mockery and disparagement. The elements are self-explanatory.

When Christine Boden (1998) first received her diagnosis of dementia, she said it felt like someone had 'pointed the bone' at her. She suddenly felt different, and that she was not a normal person any more. She spoke of going from the responsibilities of a high-level position in the public service to becoming an empty shell. This was a combination of the impact of her diagnosis and the attitudes of those around her as they responded to her diagnosis. Stokes (2010) has written of the underlying attitudes towards those who have dementia, which drives many of the responses to these people. He sees so much of the behaviour of people with dementia is attributed to the disease of dementia:

> Too often the tragic fate of people with dementia is that once they have been diagnosed with dementia everything that happens after the diagnosis is attributed to the diagnosis! Not just the dissolution of memory and intelligence but everything the person does. The pursuit of 'why' is rendered redundant, for the answer is already known – 'it is because they have dementia'. This is rarely so. Yet it is not simply because families assert that this is not their loved one that too many professionals are seduced by the simplicity of the disease model. It is also because the person is nothing like 'normal' people – they smear faeces, 'eat' inedible objects, expose themselves in front of others, hit people for no reason. People do not do such things. The result is that their behavior places them outside the human constituency, and the 'disease model' finds a receptive audience. (Stokes 2010, p.79)

In one story Stokes shared, he remarked on the importance of looking at the person, and asking relevant questions, instead of simply asserting that the disease is the reason for their behaviour. In the story of Janet, her behaviour could have been traced to her earlier life; Janet had always lived at home with her mother until her mother died. So what was the question that Janet should have been asked? It was simply, 'Why had Janet never left home?' If that question had been asked, they would have found out that Janet had always been shy and insecure. The behaviour that she exhibited while trying to cope in this strange environment that she could not understand, as a person with dementia, was consistent with her past history (Stokes 2010).

Other ethical principles

We have already considered autonomy in dementia and noted its inability to address some important issues for these vulnerable people. Three other ethical principles may also be applied within dementia care: beneficence and non-maleficence may guide doing 'good' and not harming the person with dementia; remembering too that there are others in relationship with the person with dementia as well – their family and care providers. The fourth and final accepted bioethical principle, first introduced by Beauchamp and Childress (1979), is that of justice. The focus of use of these ethical principles was built on the idea of identifying and solving a dilemma.

In the context of aged care, the decision-maker is the client, so long as the client is deemed to be competent. These concepts have largely driven ethical decision-making in health and aged care since their introduction several decades ago (Holstein, Parks and Waymack 2011). Holstein *et al.* note the apparent difficulties that the practice of these principles incurred in aged care settings. These difficulties related to family members, professional staff and the disabilities and losses experienced by older people associated with the ageing process. Although the principles and rules associated with them gave a framework for decision-making, in practice decisions were not easily made along these lines. They note also, and importantly, the context from which the principles themselves emerged: an American context, with its strong emphasis on individualism and autonomy, which may not be relevant in other cultural environments. At the core of these principles lay the concept of free choice of the client. Among some older people, the exercise of these principles was bound to encounter difficulties; if the person could not freely choose, then what? Who could choose? What would they choose and why? What responsibilities for making 'right' choices would fall to those who became the surrogate decision-makers? What would happen in the cases where there were numbers of conflicting decision-makers, or none? In the context of dementia, it also seems important to consider the other players in relationship with the person who has dementia. What about them and their characteristics that might be important in ethical decision-making and people with dementia?

The practice of the virtues in dementia care

We have asserted that the person with dementia may be vulnerable, especially as their cognitive function deteriorates. It is then that virtue ethics gain greater importance. The relationship between the person in need of care and the care provider is an important one to acknowledge. Virtue ethics consider the characteristics of the agent, or the care provider, that lead the person to consistently act in ways that are just or virtuous. Pellegrino and Thomasma (1993) argue that the 'moral essence of a health profession is the special relationship that sickness and the response to illness creates between healer and the patient' (p.xii). A similar relationship can be seen for the pastoral care provider. The challenges of providing sensitive and appropriate care can only be met by carers who believe that continuing to care and give appropriate care is important, simply because it is needed. Often the rewards for effective care are not received by those who care. It is hard to consistently provide good care for a person who may not be able to respond to the given care, who may not be able even to say 'thank you', who may not be able to speak at all or who responds inappropriately. Some care providers seem to have an innate ability to continue to respond effectively to residents who have complex needs; these abilities may be fostered and enhanced through education, but there is also something quite intrinsic about the type of caring that is required. Care of the person with advanced dementia calls forth the most highly skilled care from the carer. We suggest that it is only the person who has that capacity to work virtuously, that is, within the framework of virtue ethics, who will be able to deliver this care.

Concepts of burden of care versus privilege of care

Even the way in which we use the language of dementia has ethical implications. Often the experience of caring for people who have dementia is couched in terms of 'burden'. Surveys are more likely to ask questions about the experience of burden than of growth experience. Much of the publicity on dementia in recent years has focused on lack of cure and resultant hopelessness for those who have the disease. Lichtenberg (2009), in his editorial, clearly outlined the prevailing picture. In this article he outlined the confusion that surrounds numbers of publications on dementia and the fear generated among patients, families, health professionals and researchers. The words used in surveys are often emotive and may focus on one side only of the experience. What happens if the questions are broadened to ask about the positive experiences of caring for a loved one who has dementia?

Netto, Goh and Yap (2009) have taken a broader view of caring in a qualitative study to examine caregiver responses associated with what they have learnt and how they have grown through the experiences of caregiving. They believe that this approach has enabled caregivers to see their experience more as life-giving, rather than life-sapping, and even as a privilege.

The media, healthcare providers and researchers among others can influence the story that becomes the way in which dementia is seen by the community and hence by patients and their families. These are the attitudes and the context that influence the study participants and those who care for them. These are the stories that prevail within the community. Thus when a project is conducted that seeks to assist people with dementia to find meaning through engaging them in spiritual reminiscence, these attitudes will be a background to the conduct of the study. This will influence the way in which any of the players can see the possibilities or otherwise for change.

Vulnerability issues in conducting research with people who have dementia

We have already spoken about the vulnerability of people with dementia. When planning a research project with people who have dementia, this potential for vulnerability becomes an important area for concern. At first glance, it might not seem appropriate to have people with dementia in research studies, but the very need to give them a voice and improve quality of life means that research is of vital importance. The people we wish to study are deemed to be vulnerable, and therefore should be protected from anything that would compromise their well-being. Obviously, the benefits of being involved in research must be weighed against the risks to the person. Before ethics approval can be given for research to be conducted with people who have dementia, it must be shown that any potential risks can be overcome or prevented. It is not enough to say these people are not able to give consent and therefore research can only be conducted with the consent of their next of kin. This is to disregard the personhood of the one with dementia. There is often also debate about whether a person with dementia can give informed consent to participate in research. So, in practice, how do we go about obtaining informed consent and protecting these vulnerable people in the process of research?

It is only in the past couple of decades that people with dementia have been considered as research participants. Prior to that time, ethics committees would be likely to question the validity of any research that sought to interview or conduct surveys of people with dementia, either regarding them as unreliable witnesses, or incapable of being able to understand questions or give meaningful responses. Following on from Kitwood's (1997) vital work, Woods (1999), commenting on the substantial amount of research coming out of care-provider literature, and the contrasting paucity of research and literature on people with dementia, wrote:

> When the perspective of a person with dementia is seriously addressed, it emerges that it is not always necessary for another to speak on that person's behalf. When questions are asked carefully, thoughtfully, and sensitively, answers are not haphazard or random. They show consistency during the interview and over time. (p.35)

This has to some extent been addressed, certainly within the development of person-centred care. But still too many assumptions of the 'missing person' colour the research and care environment. These are basic issues of ethics in relation to those with mental illness.

Issues to consider prior to deciding to involve people with dementia as research participants

It remains important to ask this first question: Is it ethical to include people with dementia in research? The answer depends on a number of factors addressed below. These are vulnerable people and could be coerced into participating. They could be 'unreliable' participants, due to inability to communicate clearly, or to understand questions; therefore data obtained from them may be misleading. They could become anxious due to questioning. This, we think, is an area that needs careful consideration. A number of factors are to be considered:

1. The purpose of the research must be judged to be of potential real benefit to the participants. We cannot be certain of the exact outcomes of a particular study, but we must be able to see that there could be potential benefit for the participants. It is noted that if we were 100 per cent sure of what we would find in a research project, it is unlikely that there would be sound reason to do it.

2. A growing body of anecdotal evidence has emerged over the past two decades to show that person-centred care provides valuable support and quality of care for these people. However, anecdotal evidence alone is not enough to build best practice on.

Further testing of this evidence is needed, so that evidence-based care practices can be instituted. It would be unethical to deny new care practices on the basis of being unable to study the effects of the proposed interventions.

3. Best research in the field of dementia is research that does not foreclose on possibilities, so that new theory and practice can be developed; thus qualitative methods are important in these early stages of development. At the same time, these should be combined with quantitative methods. So effective research methods will mostly be mixed-methods study. The qualitative methods will allow exploration of themes and issues of interest previously unexamined; quantitative measures will show the effectiveness of care.

4. We cannot provide evidence-based practice in dementia care without doing the study to determine what works best for these people. The benefits of including these people as participants must outweigh any detrimental effects, such as fear, anxiety, increasing confusion and behaviour problems.

5. Obtaining consent must be done in a way that honours and protects these people, and they must be given the benefit of the doubt in being able to understand the explanations and to be asked to sign to give consent. This will be further explained, with examples from research, below.

6. All proposed research must be examined and approved according to the guidelines laid down by national bodies that govern research standards. In Australia, the National Health and Medical Research Council (NHMRC) has set out clear guidelines based on internationally agreed standards of ethical conduct for research (NHMRC 2007). Each university and each organisation that conducts research or has research studies conducted in their organisation is required to examine and approve each proposed study.

Issues about consent
Who gives consent for participation in research projects?
An approach that regards the person with dementia as an object, unable to give consent, will result in failure to ask the person with dementia for consent in a research project. In a number of situations, the legal guardian is the person approached to give consent. However, we believe it is vital to include

the person with dementia in all decisions about them and their care, even if it may seem that they do not really understand what is going on. Decisions to include or exclude people from decision-making, based on assumptions of other people regarding their cognitive status, may be inappropriate, and we believe it is best practice always to affirm the person with dementia, by inviting them to give consent and including them in all aspects of care. This is simply a measure of respect for the dignity of the human being. The safety clause is that we would also require consent from the legal guardian of the person, if the person with dementia is in residential care.

It was interesting that, in some facilities that we visited, staff appeared to have difficulty in understanding these requirements. More than once, when our research staff went to collect the signed forms, they were only given forms from the family or guardians, but no consent had been obtained from the residents who were to participate. When asked why there were no forms from the prospective study participants, the response was invariably, 'But there was no point in asking the residents, because they wouldn't know what they were signing.' The assumption was made on the side of incompetence, not competence. These assumptions are made on the basis of the care provider's understanding of the nature of the person with dementia; hence, this is an ethical issue. In these cases we would not include these people in the study, unless their consent could be obtained. We also worked on the basis that if either party, resident or family, did not sign, then we would not include the person in the study.

Dementia denial as a barrier to research participation

When we began collecting consents for these studies, in one aged care facility, we wished to include all of the residents of a new low-care facility that was a dementia-specific unit. Letters were duly distributed with explanations, and presently a few consents were received from residents of the new unit. From that aged care facility as a whole, we only received consents from families of those who were bedbound and would be unable to physically or cognitively engage in small group work. This raised some questions about willingness to participate in research. As a result, the research staff discussed the issue of non-consent with the staff who had been responsible for collecting consents. It seemed that none of the people from this one new dementia-specific unit had wanted their relative to take part in the study. It was suggested that it might be useful for the researcher to meet with a couple of those families, if they were willing to meet, who did not give consent, to see their reasons. This was arranged, and during conversation it emerged that the problem was that family members did not want their loved one 'to know they had dementia' – such is the stigma of dementia. Through discussion it became evident that family members would have readily agreed to give consent had the term 'memory loss' been substituted for 'dementia' in the letters of information and consent. We did amend our information and consent letters to reflect this finding.

Providing participants with appropriate experiences within the research process

It is important that the content of projects has meaning to the participants; this is probably even more important to consider when working with people who have dementia. We have found that people with dementia responded to meaningful activities. Finding meaning in the face of ageing, loss, disability and dementia is critical to human well-being and flourishing (Frankl 1984). Lesser (2006) notes that, even in severe dementia, self-awareness may be damaged but identity is not destroyed. Murphy (2006) maintains that memory does not truly capture all of what is required to secure personal identity. It could be argued that memory, and maybe anticipation, rationality and intellectual and political capacities, may be missing to various degrees, but what remains in the person with dementia is important: self-awareness, self-transcendence, creativity, moral capacity and perhaps social, aesthetic and religious capacities. These latter capacities are all associated with emotional and spiritual aspects of being human.

Through the many in-depth interviews and small group sessions we have conducted, it is apparent that memory loss and dementia are spoken about by some but not by others. So, as the stigma of dementia remains, this is an area for sensitivity in relation to questions and discussion. It would be good, however, for people to be able to speak openly about dementia. Perhaps further research may be a means of this occurring, particularly as research becomes translated into practice and is more widely known. More people seem to be willing to speak of their dementia, and the number of books now being published by people who have dementia is helping to break down this stigma.

End-of-life issues for people with dementia

Dementia (including Alzheimer's disease) is the third most common cause of death for older females (8.5%) and the sixth for older males (4.5%)

(Australian Institute of Health and Welfare 2010). In the UK dementia and related diseases were placed in the top ten causes of death (National End of Life Care Intelligence Network 2010). As dementia will at some point lead to death, albeit that death may be from some other cause, end-of-life issues are important for people with dementia. Because of complications around dementia and the very vulnerability of people with dementia, ethical issues are particularly important. Issues that are likely to arise relate to diagnosis and disclosure of diagnosis (Sullivan and O'Conor 2001), feeding when no longer capable of swallowing, pain relief and communication challenges (MacKinlay 2006).

To disclose or withhold diagnosis to the person with dementia has been much discussed. It is apparent that in many cases the person does know, or at least suspect, the diagnosis, and sometimes a conspiracy of silence lies between the person, their family and care providers. Like talking about death, unless dementia is a topic that can be spoken of, people will often be reluctant to raise it. Christine Bryden (Boden) found that, after the initial shock, it was helpful for her to know her diagnosis (MacKinlay 2006, 2011). She suffered from depression in the early months following her diagnosis, and it is hard to say whether this may have been related to disclosure of the diagnosis in any way. However, knowing, rather than just suspecting, the diagnosis did enable Christine to plan for her future. Importantly, it allowed the diagnosis to be on the table – we exposed the 'elephant in the room'. We were able to speak of it openly, and this in itself seemed to be a powerful enabler. One of the issues, of course, about disclosure and speaking of dementia, is to be able to traverse the barriers within other people who hold the myths of the 'non-person'. It may be very confronting to such people to have to interact with people who have dementia.

Refusal to accept treatment

Concern was raised by Lotty (below) about the consequences of a resident or patient refusing treatment. There are misunderstandings about such decisions, for instance that refusal of treatment does not mean that the person is abandoned. Care moves then from curative to palliative care, which of course includes effective pain management.

Facilitator: The hardest things for you now?

Lotty: Except that I, well I mean my life is over virtually. I mean mentally I need that, I, well I can't do, well I have done a lot of hard work, I mean I can't even nurse a baby any more, I'd drop it. I think that I'm, if I can express it, I would rather they hadn't saved my life in my last illness, but you're in a point these days where you are, you can refuse treatment, which I did, but they get back at you because they don't give you any relief from pain.

Facilitator: Oh now that shouldn't happen. You should never ever be denied relief from pain.

Lotty: Well that is what is done in the hospital these days.

Advance directives are also important in setting the scene for the end-of-life process for people who have dementia. These issues have been dealt with in other publications (MacKinlay 2006); this book focuses more on the person and their life-meaning.

Summary

This chapter has explored issues related to identity of the person in dementia and the ethical implications of our attitudes towards those with dementia. It has examined issues of vulnerability and autonomy, highlighting the need to consider interdependency as the true goal for humans, rather than autonomy. The importance of virtue ethics has shown the requirements for the care provider to become self-aware and inculcate the traits of a virtuous person; not subservient, but being truthful, humble, gentle and sensitive to the person with dementia. End-of-life issues, as relevant to this topic, have been explored in the context of ethical issues around dying and death; however, death is such an important topic that we have devoted a separate chapter to it.

5

Resilience and Transcendence

One of the spiritual tasks of ageing identified by MacKinlay (2001a) is transcendence. It involves being able to self-forget and move beyond concern for oneself, to reach out to others. This task of ageing is also associated with meaning. What might the experience of meaning and transcendence in later life be for people with dementia? First, it is useful to consider the wider field, that of meaning and transcendence in cognitively competent older people.

The process of physical and psychosocial ageing and transcendence

An exploration of psychosocial ageing and the spiritual process of transcendence must include consideration of our attitudes towards both ageing and the natural culmination of the life journey – death. Jones (2001) has clearly articulated Western societal attitudes and values regarding older people:

> The aging person, ailing and pitiful, becomes a symbol for our common fate: death. To avoid the reality of our own death, we simply corral and avoid the elderly. While in Puritan days death was viewed as a glorious reunion, a birthing into eternity, it is the denial of death that marks heavily our society. (Jones 2001, p.102)

This may be the outcome of the ageing process, if the possibilities for spiritual growth that are potentially possible for older adults are neglected. Harris (2008), writing of the possibilities of spiritual growth at the end of life, suggests that it is not only the relevance of spiritual resources that people have when they reach these critical points of life, but that the very experience of facing the end of life may stimulate growth and development of spiritual resources not previously held. In fact, Harris writes of the potential for spiritual formation in this last time of life. Harris has suggested that the experience of dying may not be so difficult, when in the process of dying we can discover who we are. MacKinlay (2006) has also recorded the importance of this final stage of life and journey towards death. Later life, increasing frailty and chronic illness can bring a raised awareness of our mortality to us, which can be the starting point for spiritual growth.

Transcendence in later life

In this publication, the word *transcendence* is used to describe a situation where the person moves beyond self-centredness to other-centredness. This is an important aspect of Erikson's psychosocial stages of ageing, where the eighth stage is seen as integrity versus despair. This construct has been studied in relation to the spiritual dimension in ageing, and described by MacKinlay (2001a, 2001b) in the spiritual model of themes and the model of the tasks and process of ageing (see chapter 1).

An important aspect of this ageing journey, it seems, is to learn how to transcend the naturally occurring losses and disabilities that so often accompany the ageing process. A brief consideration of related literature in trauma experiences may be helpful in understanding the possibilities for spiritual and emotional growth in the face of increasing disability. Recent paradigms of trauma experience have often been couched in terms of loss and suffering (Vis and Boynton 2008), where the so-called 'survivors' are left with only the negative views rather than a full range of possibilities that might also include growth and transcendence of the trauma. The authors, researching within a framework of social work, have taken an alternative approach, to examine spiritual growth and transcendence in the experience of loss and trauma, moving towards meaning making, noting that they believe that 'spirituality is an extension of worldview, coping, and meaning making, and is an essential component in healthy posttraumatic processing' (Vis and Boynton 2008, p.70). While this study focuses on a study of spirituality in post-trauma events, it is postulated that it also be of relevance in understanding the process of growing older and the events that may surround that, which not uncommonly include major losses and disabilities. Albeit that these do not usually come into the definition of trauma, they may still be perceived as being traumatic by those who experience them.

According to Vis and Boynton (2008) a traumatic event 'is often described as an unexpected stress-related event that produces intense feelings of fear, anxiety, or helplessness' (p.70). These are certainly some of the experiences of older people as they face significant losses and disabilities. Some may be foreseen, but other events come unexpectedly and suddenly. The focus taken by Vis and Boynton is the potential for growth in the post-trauma event, suggesting that the major effect of the event is to challenge the person's world-view and life-meaning. They see opportunities for reintegration of the person's meaning into a new world-view that may offer hope. Their view fits well with the view of ageing and loss, where story or narrative can be used, especially in the spiritual dimension to connect with meaning and a reframing of world-view to incorporate aspects of growth and meaning making and the associated transcendence (MacKinlay 2006). Vis and Boynton (2008) go so far as to say that '[i]nformation that is processed during meaning formation post-trauma cannot escape spiritual reflection' (p.74).

Taking the model of spiritual growth and care (MacKinlay 2006), the process of transcendence and transformation can be seen where loss may challenge life-meaning and stimulate the search for new meaning (see Figure 5.1). Where new meaning is not found, despair may result. The process of coming to new meanings is started through the personal sense of vulnerability that is often present among older adults, especially those moving into frailty. Their vulnerability is realised through actual loss and disability, and this may shake and weaken previous life-meanings; several older people have shared personal experiences[1] of an increased sense of life as precarious as they have become frailer. This presents challenges for the older vulnerable person – Can they incorporate these experiences in their life story? Do these experiences enable hope? If hope cannot be seen, then the alternative of despair may become the new life focus. Thus, the very losses and disabilities experienced in later life may be life-giving or life-constricting.

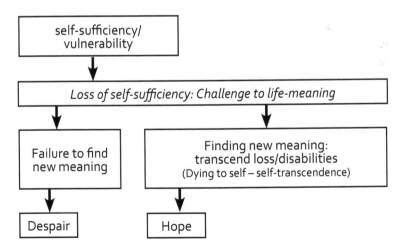

Figure 5.1 *A process of self-transcendence in later life*

---

1   Personal communications with Elizabeth MacKinlay.

In fact, the topic of transcendence and spiritual formation is not a new topic. It has been known at least since the Middle Ages. The works of St Francis (Nicholson 1923; Sabatier 2003) and others of the mystics of that time show abundant evidence of the awareness and practices of spiritual disciplines that had an intentional goal of self-transcendence. For St Francis, it was a continuing journey of growing into deeper relationship with God, seeking, as others of the mystics have done before and since, to grow into union with God. St Francis did not live a long life, being only about 44 years of age when he died; however, the manner of his living of intentional seeking after transformation into Christ has set a model of transcendence that many have endeavoured to emulate in the centuries since his life in the 13th century. It is interesting that his model, set so long ago, still retains relevance today. St Francis actually established three orders: two enclosed and one in which members remained living in the world within their everyday occupations but sought to live their lives under a simple rule that focused on others and God, and not on the material aspects of life. For many people, the way of St Francis may seem hard; living lives modelled on Christ and focusing on humility, poverty, simplicity, chastity, love and joy. And yet, these things are essential means of becoming really alive, and can be used in fostering ways of transcending the disabilities and losses that naturally occur in later life. It is suspected that these might be a means of moving towards the transcendence that seems to come naturally to some older people.

How can 21st-century people tap into these tested modes of spiritual growth and development? In largely secular Western societies this can be challenging, as fewer people have connections with a religious faith that might provide guidance in spiritual growth. However, if we consider the universal nature of the spiritual dimension, being potentially present in all people and therefore to be regarded as part of being human, then it seems to be worthwhile assessing ways of developing spiritual strengths for older people, both those who practise a religious faith and those who do not. Work of relevance to this field is that of Erikson, Erikson and Kivnick (1986) in the well-known psychosocial stages of ageing, where the eighth stage was integrity versus despair. This stage is viewed as an important time when people can review their lives and revisit earlier stages of psychosocial development and rework issues from earlier developmental stages. Erikson has said that this stage potentially has an outcome of wisdom. This eighth stage can also be regarded as a spiritual stage, of coming to a realisation of spiritual integrity, and the wisdom that may accompany this development. MacKinlay (2001a) has developed a definition of spiritual integrity, based on the study of in-depth interviews of older people:

A state where an individual shows by their life example and attitudes, a sense of peace within themselves and others, and development of wholeness of being. The search for meaning and a degree of transcendence is evident. (p.180)

At that time, it was noted that 'true wholeness and integrity is probably only possible at the point of death[;] however, many may approach it in the later stages of life' (MacKinlay 2001a, p.180). As previously mentioned, some frail older people have described the life journey as becoming 'more precarious'. This can be understood through Erikson's stages as the journey into wisdom. Taking this further, to explore the spiritual dimension, a spiritual context of wisdom can be defined as:

An increased tolerance to uncertainty, a deepening search for meaning in life, including an awareness of the paradoxical and contradictory nature of reality; it involves transcendence of uncertainty and a move from external to internal regulation. (MacKinlay 2001a, p.153)

Therefore this may indeed be a journey into wisdom, if wisdom is defined within a spiritual context. Another term that has found popularity recently is *resilience*. What is meant by the term? Generally it means to be hardy, or to be able to survive in difficult circumstances. Resilience is the ability to rise above stress, loss, adversity or disability. We may also see older people who can be said to be flourishing; which is about living life to the full, without reservations, and perhaps even being willing to take risks, where the benefits of taking the risks can be seen to outweigh the consequences of the risks. On the other hand, could it be that a person with dementia may be more likely to take a risk without seeming to fully understand the consequences? Resilience and flourishing are both aspects of transcendence. The person who is on the way to transcendence may have a sense of freedom and see possibilities open for new ways of being.

Gerotranscendence

The dominant social theory that has driven policy and practice in aged care in recent decades has been activity theory, with emphasis given to engaging older people in activities within residential aged care. However, more recently, a new concept has emerged, that of gerotranscendence; this new concept has gone back to recapture the earlier stage of theory development in social gerontology. It is based on Cumming and Henry's (1961) theory of disengagement, where older people disengage from the roles of mid-life and become more reflective as they grow older. It is likely that this is associated with the development of frailty.

Lars Tornstam (1999/2000, 2005) was responsible for establishing the importance of the concept of gerotranscendence as a life stage of the latter part of life, having taken up the largely neglected concepts of disengagement theory (Cumming and Henry 1961) to show that some disengagement does occur in the frailty of later life, especially among those who, due to frailty, have lower energy levels and are facing their final life career. This is an important discovery and is relevant for care policy and practice in residential aged care, where in recent years activity theory has been the driving force that underlies policy, programmes and care. This also fits with Rick Moody's (1995) description of ageing 'being like a natural monastery', in that older people may become more reflective and introspective. Older people who no longer have the energy to be engaged with many activities may have other 'work' to do, the work of coming to a sense of their final life-meanings, and the process of self-transcendence that accompanies this process.

Exploring meaning in later life, a process of spiritual reminiscence

The small spiritual reminiscence groups provided a place where all have been able to share their life experiences and the place of meaning in their lives whether or not they had a religious faith.

In the spiritual tasks and process of ageing model (MacKinlay 2001a, 2001b) one of the tasks is to work through the struggle of the losses and vulnerabilities of later life, and to come to a sense of transcendence through this struggle. In earlier work (MacKinlay 2001a) it was often the person who had experienced crises and significant losses in their lives who managed to grow most spiritually, in these later years. Of course this was not always so, and some who experienced significant loss, even the loss of a life partner, seemed to become blocked in their spiritual development. From the data of these earlier studies, this journey to find transcendence seemed to be an important task of ageing. In fact it is also associated with the development of hope and the finding of final life meanings as well (see Figure 1.3 in Chapter 1).

A basic first step along this road to transcendence, or, as Frankl (1984) termed it, self-forgetting, is to be able to accept and live with the losses and disabilities of everyday life. The journey to self-transcendence begins as the person realises their vulnerability, and recognises that they are unable to retain self-sufficiency and autonomy. Fear often emerges at this stage. An elderly woman living in the UK who had severe arthritis recently travelled to Switzerland for assisted suicide as she reportedly did not wish to 'dwindle away', and wished to go, that is, to die, at a time of her own choosing.[2] It seems so sad that the struggles of later life might lead to such termination of life, where there seems to be nothing to live for if perfect health is no longer possible. Coupled with this is a perceived lack of availability of care for the person in need, and unwillingness to burden others. Still others find a different way, through a path of struggle to transcendence and resilience. Does being able to share and journey with other older people help in developing transcendence? At this stage, we do not have a great deal of evidence on this topic; what we do know is that spiritual reminiscence can be very affirming for those who take part in this process. This major study has explored and examined the process of spiritual reminiscence with people who have dementia.

Concepts of positive or successful ageing and dementia

Often emphasis is placed on positive or successful ageing, and in this context it cannot really be said that people with dementia are ageing successfully. Perhaps in this context, it could be said that they had failed the test of ageing – but have they? It all depends on how ageing is defined. If ageing is defined purely in biological and psychological parameters, then people with dementia will probably fail the mental health test, although they might pass on the physical health test. But is this all that growing older is about? Jones (2001) writes of the three marks of success in Western societies: power, status and security. To some extent, all of these are lost during the process of ageing, and this is particularly so in dementia.

So far, in this chapter, we have focused on transcendence and transformation among cognitively competent people. But as the focus of this book is on people who have dementia, we turn next to the findings from our work with people who have dementia. The process of growing older and also having dementia may seem to be just 'too much'. The process of ageing itself is often regarded negatively, so being diagnosed with dementia as well may be just too hard.

---

2 As widely reported in the UK daily press in April 2011.

Transcendence in later life and dementia

While self-transcendence is understood as a process that numbers of older people experience to a greater or lesser extent, transcendence among people with dementia is relatively unstudied and thus unknown. But can transcendence be present in people who have dementia?

By using this model in the study of finding meaning in dementia, through the process of spiritual reminiscence, it was possible to examine the words of the participants, both in their initial in-depth interviews and in the subsequent small group sessions over either the short six-week groups or the longer 24-week groups. We will examine the data for examples of transcendence and also for examples of lack of transcendence.

Gerotranscendence in dementia

The concept of gerotranscendence (Tornstam 1999/2000, 2005) as a means of considering ageing and dementia may provide a valuable new lens for viewing the person with dementia. Tornstam has identified a process of disengagement, increasing reflection and contemplation that seems to occur in many older people as they become frailer. In the model of the spiritual tasks and process of ageing, this task is related to self-transcendence versus vulnerability. Vulnerability has been addressed most specifically in the chapter on ethical aspects of research and practice with vulnerable people. The spiritual task here is self-transcendence, or in the words of Frankl (1984), the process of self-forgetting, or to use Christian, Pauline terms, to die to self. It involves concepts of suffering, letting go and moving onwards to focus on others rather than self. Its place in dementia has been little considered. In this study it was possible to examine instances of transcendence and resilience among these people, both through the initial in-depth interviews and as they participated in the weekly small group sessions.

Self-transcendence was identified as one of the six main tasks in the process of ageing from a spiritual perspective (MacKinlay 1998, 2001a). Initial data that led to this model being developed was based on the mapping of the spiritual dimension of older independent-living people, all of whom were cognitively intact. In the study being reported in this book, the work was with people who have dementia. Common wisdom might have concluded that transcendence would not be possible for people with dementia as intact cognitive processes would be a prerequisite for transcendence to occur. Was this the case? Further, would self-transcendence that had occurred prior to the onset of dementia be protective against some or any of the disruptive behaviours that may be seen in dementia?

One of the greatest barriers to self-transcendence is fear. Fear was acknowledged by 100 per cent of the independent older people in the original study (MacKinlay 1998), as they contemplated losing their autonomy and perhaps losing control of their lives through suffering or unrelieved pain in their later days (MacKinlay 2001a). In a subsequent study of frail older people (MacKinlay 2006) only 45 per cent of participants said that they held fears for the future; while this is a large shift from the 100 per cent of independent-living older people who said they held fears for the future, it did still mean that 55 per cent of these older people held at least some fears. All of these people were already frail, and lived with more than one chronic health condition and required high-level residential care, but they were all cognitively intact. Why was there such a large change in levels of fear between the two groups? When asked, these frail participants said that what had changed for them, after being admitted to an aged care facility, was that they felt safe and secure. They felt that, if they had a need, there would be someone they could call on to help them. It is noted, however, that these were all older people who were cognitively intact; would the experience be similar for people with dementia? What levels of awareness would people with dementia actually have? Our model of the process of the spiritual tasks of ageing proved to be a valuable way of connecting with people with dementia. The process of spiritual reminiscence certainly opened the way for these people expressing their thoughts, and especially their feelings about living with dementia and growing older.

What is it like to be growing older with dementia?

But what about people who have dementia? Often we think of people with dementia as not being aware of their own life journey, let alone being able to reflect on and achieve a sense of transcendence or to be able to be resilient. So what is the experience of ageing like for these people with dementia? Might this be the same, or similar, for these people, or might it be quite different between cognitively intact and cognitively impaired older people? Is it possible that there is no meaning in the experience of dementia? Christine Bryden (Boden) shared her concern as she looked to a future of increasing cognitive impairment, due to her dementia, and asked the question of where she would find meaning in this experience of dementia.

In our process of spiritual reminiscence, we asked similar questions of the people who had dementia to those that we used with cognitively intact older people who have participated in spiritual reminiscence groups. We did this based on the fact that our focus was on a holistic approach to care, using person-centred care, but with a real aim of connecting with these people, not so much at the cognitive level, but at the emotional and spiritual levels (which we have done regardless of cognitive status). As well, we were focusing on what we knew of responses of people with dementia from previous research. This was another important reason for choosing *not* to use a highly cognitive approach. A focus on factual questions could be threatening and produce a situation where these already vulnerable people may fear failure. On the other hand, because we already knew that people with dementia can respond to questions of meaning, and emotional and spiritual aspects, we prepared work that would address this emphasis.

The questions we asked in small group sessions that were related to this task of transcendence and transformation are listed below. It is emphasised that these were very broad questions and these questions were asked by *inviting* the person to respond (see chapter 12 for processes of communication):

- What's it like growing older?
  - For example, do you have any health problems?
  - Do you have memory problems? If so, how does that affect what you want to do?
- What are the hardest things in your life now?
- Do you like living here? What's it like living here? Was it hard to settle in? (And other questions of a similar kind.)
- As you reach the end of your life, what do you hope for now?
- What do you look forward to?

A further broad question asked in the in-depth interviews, but not followed through generally in the small group sessions, was 'What are the good things in your life?'

Based on the results of the study, we would first like to share with you some responses that form a representative summary of responses of these people with dementia in the group sessions. These are direct quotations from the participants, all of whom had a diagnosis of dementia.

The exchanges below provide examples from one of the group sessions where the facilitator is simply asking older people with dementia what the experience was like for them. There is some gentle humour, some hopes, some disappointments for the future, some acceptance, and also some wisdom. The following response from an in-depth interview is light-hearted:

Interviewer: What is it like growing older?

Anita: I think it takes a while to get used to it. It's freedom. (*laughs*)

The responses from a group session are recorded below; a mixture of attitudes and ways of accepting growing older:

Daphne: You are 90?

Hetty: Yes.

Daphne: Yes.

Hetty: And I never thought I would get there.

Daphne: Mmm.

Hetty: My family, the young ones, reckon I will get to 100.

Facilitator: Get to 100?

Hetty: Yes.

Facilitator: Yes, I reckon you will.

Rose: I don't want to live to 100.

Hetty: No, I don't particularly.

Rose: You have to go the way you want to get out.

Hetty: 100.

Rose: 100, oh right.

Facilitator: It's a high number, isn't it?

Daphne: I think it is true for most of us, that as we get older we get weaker, in one way or another. Some people cannot hear, some can't see, some can't walk, all those sorts of things beset us, which we have not experienced before, because we can always do plenty just when and where we like. Can't do it any more, dependent upon somebody else very often.

Facilitator: Mmm. Somebody else's eyes, or somebody else's ears, or somebody else's hands. Is that right?

As can be seen in the exchanges above, participant responses were in many ways similar to the kinds of responses that we might have expected from cognitively intact people. If we had asked factual questions, it is likely that the responses would not have been nearly so fruitful. One area that borders between normal ageing and dementia is the topic of memory loss. The same group discussed their experiences of growing older and memory loss:

Facilitator: What do you think, Ben, are you enjoying old age, or...?

Ben: Hardly say enjoyed, but...managing to adapt to it. Except for memory losses.

Facilitator: Yes, that must be hard to come to grips with, is it?

Ben: Yes.

Facilitator: How does it affect you?

Ben: Just kind of frustrating.

Facilitator: So, I remember you saying something to me this morning, you wanted to tell me something, you got half way through it and then you couldn't remember the next word. Do you find that that's the frustrating part?

Ben: Yes, that's the frustrating part. So you know what you want to say in your mind, but sometimes when you go to say it, it won't come.

Facilitator: Is that what happens?

Ben: I just black out.

Facilitator: Right. Do you find that, Anita? Does that happen to you sometimes?

Anita: I find that I just can't think what I want to say.

Una struggled to express herself, and acknowledged the troubles of remembering, in this excerpt; while her MMSE was 19 at the beginning of the 24-week programme, at the end of testing it was just 4. However, she was still able to make herself understood.

Una: Oh dear, I'm so old aren't I? 96 am I? I'm not sure, I might be just on 90 ,I'm not sure what age I am, in October's my birthday. Uh hm. I think I still love beer, I can't remember.

Examples of good things in life

A simple question, more often asked in the in-depth interviews than in the small groups, was: 'What are the good things in your life now?' This was a good way of inviting the participant to share how they felt about life, what the experience was like and where they were now in their life journey. This was not a threatening question (they were also asked about the hard things and about fears). For many of these older people, the view was quite positive. Many of the responses focused on family; many also focused on health. This is also interesting, as when independent-living older people are asked how they would feel about living up until 100 years or more, a typical answer is 'It all depends on my health; if I am healthy it would be fine, but I don't want to live that long if I have to suffer' – there remains a sense of fear around future suffering and pain for many people.

Some of the responses to the question about the good things now were:

Unidentified participant: My family. They are always there for me, I have two sons. And they come and see me.

Hetty: Well I had, apart from this stroke, I have had a very healthy life, I have never been very big because I have been very healthy. 'Cause my son and daughter, they had a conversation, and they decided that I was the fittest of them, them all.

Claire: Oh well I suppose getting married and having my daughter, things like, things that normally happen.

Daphne: Just thinking about the future, and the future for me, is to go and, uh, at one time, when he is ready, uh, put me into, um, a place that he has prepared for me.

Facilitator: Yes.

Daphne: And this is really my whole heart, the other is just struggling along, as you will find most of us are. We struggle along, some better than others, and my hearing is quite good, my sight is awful, I can hardly see anything, and my walking is awful, I can't do very much, but I still manage to go out on the bus, and that affords some relief, some different atmosphere, so to speak, and as long as I get that to walk here, in here, that sort of, hasn't got wheels on it, you will see, just slides along, so it's not suitable to take outside, but as long as I can get to the bus stop which is just across the road.

...

Daphne: So I manage very well, but um, when you say what is the greatest thing,[3] *in a way there is not anything on earth because I just think that my journey is almost to the end, and I am hoping it is*, uh, not, not, I was depressed last week, not very often I am, but what with the kitchen and everything else all being out of order, and everybody being at their wit's end, and not knowing what what's where, and it's, um, I do feel, a lot better this week, and I have got back to normal again now.

The participant in the exchange above came back to the original question (of the good things in life) some time later, and reflected on her life journey. She seemed to be looking to life after death in the comment above in italics.

---

3   The participant here is responding to an earlier question. It was not uncommon for people with cognitive disabilities to take some time to start to answer a question. In fact it was only in looking back at the transcripts that you could sometimes see that they were responding appropriately, but to an earlier question, well passed by in the conversation.

Louise, who had an MMSE score of only 4, when asked about the good things in life, responded as follows:

Louise: Oh, well I don't know because I am used to now, being here, and you know everybody popping in and out.

Interviewer: Yes, and being here is good?

Louise: Pardon?

Interviewer: Being here is good?

Louise: Well it is to me, I mean now, I don't know what really.

Relationship was important and classed as one of the good things for Bronwyn, while health was important for John:

Facilitator: What are the good things in your life now?

Bronwyn: To be here, which I really enjoy, and to be with my husband and my family as long as I can.

John: The best thing in my life now? Oh it would be the continuation of reasonably good health, because after all I am starting to wind down.

Facilitator: Hmm.

John: And err, the kids to progress and the grandkids grow up and that.

Facilitator: Yeah.

John: And the continuity of a moderate life whereby we try to maintain a level of what would you say? Um, good living.

Facilitator: Yes.

John: With good living goes the fact that you should err be moderate in everything you do. Other than that, oh and good health goes hand in hand with you.

Examples of transcendence in the transcripts

Good things were sometimes complex combinations of good and difficult experiences. It seemed that these people with cognitive difficulties would speak of what was of central importance to them, which might not have been in a category of 'good experiences' as in the example below, where tragedy seemed to mix with strength and with the recognition that transcendence is possible.

Interviewer: What are the good things in your life now?

Eunice: The good things in my life. There's um, um this place here, um she got me in here, the doctor couldn't but she did. Um good things in my life, ah my Grandson committed suicide a fortnight ago, he was 45.

Interviewer: That is so, so sad.

Eunice: She's had a. My daughter's had a very, very hard life. A very hard life, ah I think that's why I, I'm so much her way, she's got more guts than anyone I know, never complains, never think that she's had a hard life, she's had a terrible life.

Interviewer: Oh that's sad.

Eunice: It would take you a week to listen to her life if I told you. I mean I grabbed her and her two children and ran with them and hid them and so forth, and started them off in a college education and bought a house for them. Sold my two blocks of land, that kind of life love, but it doesn't show so that's all right, I've never told them here. You don't tell people these things; they don't want to hear it.

Interviewer: No. No, I think that happens sometimes. Yeah.

Eunice: People don't want to hear that kind of thing.

Interviewer: Ah. Yeah. So we were talking about the good things in life, and we got onto...

Eunice: The good things in life. The good things in life. Well I, all life's been good to me once I married at 18, 'cause I had a hell of a childhood. I was bashed every day of my life, so there you are, and I met a man who had had a rough life, been married and raised two lovely kids.

Interviewer: And it was a good marriage?

Eunice: A lovely marriage.

Interviewer: Wow. That's wonderful. So you broke the cycle there of your own childhood.

Eunice: 18. Yes. I worked at night time with police protection, and we earned the money to buy a block of land on the Parramatta River, and we paid 250 pounds for it and took us eight years to build a house on it, the both of us built it, never borrowed money, and it sold for one million dollars two years ago, it sold for one million dollars, but we didn't own it then, we sold it for 20,000 dollars and it bought us a home up the coast. It's how I've lived. I've lived. So I'm a month off 90.

Often connections between good experiences and difficult ones can be close and intermingled; for instance, all can be going well when suddenly a change in health, a sudden onset of illness or an accident can throw up the spectre of vulnerability for the person, as in the following account:

> **Interviewer:** Can you tell me what have been the good things in your life that you can remember, what have been the good times?
>
> **Dorothy:** Well that depends on what you would call a good life and everything else.
>
> **Interviewer:** Mmm hmm.
>
> **Dorothy:** Because we were on the farm, my husband worked on the shire, and during the war he was a sleeper cutter.
>
> **Interviewer:** Very hard work.
>
> **Dorothy:** Yes. And then I was there involved with the senior cits, and had all my friends around me. So, and then I fell and shattered my arm and that shattered my world.
>
> **Interviewer:** Hmm.

The topic of 'What was it like growing older?' was discussed at length in the group sessions, and below is one example of how one small group handled issues of transcendence within the group.

> **Facilitator:** How about you, Ben, do you have aches and pains now that you didn't have when you were a younger man, or are you still okay?
>
> **Ben:** As far as aches and pains are concerned, there's no great problems.
>
> **Facilitator:** Still fairly fit?
>
> **Ben:** Reasonably fit, yes. Except for the odd fall.
>
> **Facilitator:** You fall occasionally don't you? I think you probably get up too quickly and you fall.
>
> **Ben:** No, I'm not aware of that.

The hard things of life

The questions of hard things are equally important to ask. Everyday life has both positive and negative experiences, and both should be explored. Therefore the questions here focused on the hardest things. We did not specifically name hard things, just as we did not name the 'good things', but rather left it to the participants to respond in whichever way they felt was relevant to them at that time. The hard things ranged through memory loss, not being able to do all they wanted to do, living with the disabilities produced by a stroke, missing family, and loneliness. The hard things were but one side of the coin; the other side was how these people lived with the hard things. In the exchanges reported below, we have only given examples of the hard things, not the outcomes of loss.

Facilitator: What are the hardest things in your life now? What do you find that is hard?

Anita: Oh, be interested enough to cover everything. (*laughs*)

Facilitator: So in other words, so you still want to be involved in things, but you can't.

Anita: Can't follow it all. Or else you could go, go somewhere else. I should recollect having all these feelings, you just go along and see what's happening.

Facilitator: What about you, Ben, is there anything in your life that you're finding difficult or hard at the moment?

Ben: Specific memory loss lapses.

Facilitator: How do you feel about living here?

Anita: It becomes very tiresome, it goes on and on and on, and you'd like to get out, into the world.

Facilitator: Yes, so what do you find are the hardest things in life for you now?

Amy: Losing my music, without a doubt.

Facilitator: Okay, what would you say are the hardest things in your life right now? What are the hardest things in your life right now?

Hetty: Having the stroke. I did not expect that.

Facilitator: Uh huh. How long ago did you have the stroke?

Hetty: Not sure. I am not sure.

Facilitator: The hardest things for you now?

Margaret: Oh well there's nothing very hard now. I'm settled in here, and I think I'm going along all right.

Mary: Um learning to cope with my new life.

Facilitator: So what's the hardest thing about your new life?

Mary: Not having my husband or boys around me.

Facilitator: Yeah. Are there any other hard things?

Mary: No I don't think so. I think I'm very lucky.

Karen expresses her sense of feeling alone – 'not very nice', while Sarah feels that life just continues, much the same:

Facilitator: What about you, Karen, what are the hardest things in your life now?

Karen: Well it's so; I don't know I hope I can something. But err at the moment I don't know, what is there? No, what I could say to you.

Facilitator: Do you have any difficulties?

Karen: Well yeah I'm alone.

Facilitator: You're alone?

Karen: Yeah, and that is not very nice. I thought it was, but it wasn't. So I don't know what to do.

Facilitator: What about you, Sarah, what are the hardest things in your life now? The hardest things in your life?

Sarah: Um I don't really know. I just, life just goes on the same. Um no, I don't find anything too hard, if I do a lot of my fathers, who's a very capable man and he can always help me out of a technical problem. No.

Facilitator: Violet, we talked about the breast cancer, but is there anything else that is hard for you now?

Violet: No, I keep it under control is the main thing; I know that I'll die if I can't keep that under control.

Regina identifies loneliness as being hard for her now:

Interviewer: Now, what would you say would be the hardest things in your life now?

Regina: I'm alone more. I don't like lots of people of anything, but I do feel alone at times, but I am fortunate to be the way I am.

Interviewer: Yes. Now, were you living at home before you came in here?

Regina: Um, can't remember.

Interviewer: And are you happy living here?

Regina: Yes, yes I am.

Loss of memory

Loss of memory was judged by some to be one of the hard things of growing older.

> **Interviewer:** Okay. Um, yep, I want to pick up on the question, there are a couple of things running around there. Do you want to deal with the one about memory first because you've talked about that a couple of times? Um is that a problem for you, the fact that you, you're having trouble remembering things, or is that something that you're able to accept? How do you feel about the whole thing?
>
> **Bob:** Well I can accept that. I can accept that I'm not nearly as bright as I used to be. Err whether there is ah a reasonable explanation for that I would have to say, it's age I hope.
>
> **Interviewer:** Yeah. Yeah. Why did you say 'age I hope'?
>
> **Bob:** Err, because I have unfortunately made arrangements err to remind me when I go out to dinner, and I completely forgot all about it. Whether it was after the friend that I was going out with, err a very, very lovely lad, I've known him for years. I made the thing in an attempt to go out with him for dinner and he rang me three days beforehand and said, 'So and so has cropped up, do you mind if we make it instead of Thursday if we made it for Monday of next week?' And I said, 'No, perfectly okay, we're go to dinner in Monday of next week', um that was perfectly okay, but they went, I just completely ignored him and I don't even turn up, forgotten the day and the hour. I get very embarrassed.

On the other hand, not all participants found life hard, as in the following excerpt:

> **Interviewer:** What are the hardest things in your life now?
>
> **Roslyn:** Now?
>
> **Interviewer:** Yes.
>
> **Roslyn:** Nothing, really. (*laughs*)
>
> **Interviewer:** That's great.
>
> **Roslyn:** I mean, I am keeping my will if I want to, go out and get my meals, walking down and talk to people, and we have bush trips and I always make a point of going, and you know, everything that is going, I go. I do.
>
> **Interviewer:** Stay involved.

Roslyn: No, I think I am quite fortunate to be here. I suppose sometime it does worry me that you just can't walk out of the place, you know.

Interviewer: Yes, so yeah, that would be a hard thing.

Roslyn: But when I first came, I used to go down to the shops, and so forth, and I would say well I am going out, and say that to them. But they seem to be tougher now, I don't really want to go, you know. They take us here and there, he takes us different. At 80 you don't want to be running around everywhere. (*laughs*) So I have got no regrets.

Growing older and transcendence

Transcendence is complex. The following is a conversation within one of the groups. The facilitator does just that, simply guiding the conversation. The group members engage with each other, talking about growing older. Topics discussed cover loss of different types, sadness and also affirmation and encouragement by the facilitator. It can be seen that participants acknowledge their losses and disappointments, but also talk about their acceptance of these now. For example, look at Don's contribution to the discussion, where he sees the positive side of events, and expresses feelings of hope.

Facilitator: Rose, are there things that you would like to do that you find difficult?

Rose: Yes.

Facilitator: Can you tell us some of those things?

Rose: I used to do, I love knitting, I can't do that now, I used to go out, every Friday we used to mind another mug, because my husband is dead, I have already got a daughter, and she is very good.

Facilitator: That's quite alright, Rose.

(*Rose is upset*)

...

Facilitator: Is that your daughter you're talking about?

Rose: Yes, she comes to see me.

Facilitator: You used to live in her house did you?

Rose: Yes, because after my husband died, and I was leaving the hospital, I remember she said back there, and the doctor said he was looking for a place for me, and my sister said she is not going in a place, she is coming with me, so she came over once and sold all my things, and... (*becomes emotional*)

Facilitator: Okay, Rose, thank you for sharing those very personal things, aren't they, hurtful. Lovely to have you at [name of facility]. You are such a bright spark.

Rose: I used to be. (*laughs*)

Facilitator: You are.

Rose: I used to reach, I worked with the airline, when I had a ticket to travel any airline when I wanted, so when I was retired, before I came here, I used to go everywhere, among other friends, made trips, many places.

Don: I think that is the thing that we all miss most of all.

Rose: Yes.

Don: Our independence. In the old days we could do these things for ourselves, but now we have to depend on help to do them, and that option, for a start, begins to make you feel rather sorry for yourself, and you must never let that happen, because if you look around, raise your head a bit and have a look, you will see people in a much worse condition.

Rose: Yes, there are a lot of people worse.

Don: Yes.

Facilitator: Yes, well Daphne mentioned the possibility that Hetty might like to dance.

Daphne: I used to dance.

Hetty: Can't enjoy your exercise. I can't stand on one leg, I would fall over if I stood on one and hopped the other one up, you would not have, Daphne.

Facilitator: A bit hard to balance then.

Hetty: Yes, I can assure you.

Don: When here we are, we all get together, exchanging our experiences, and that helps a lot. So, God is with us all the time, so we must enjoy our days.

This is a typical example of group interaction. For the people with dementia, the facilitator was important in setting up and establishing the group. Once the group got to know one another, they began to interact together, not only through the facilitator. They initiated conversation too.

Growing older, challenges and issues of transcendence

The excerpt below illustrates some of the tensions involved in growing frailty, the stroke, the increasing physical care and the daughter. Hetty is well aware of the added stress her daughter experiences. A stroke can be a starting point for the beginnings of transcendence, or it may simply be a point of awareness of growing dependency and depression. Hetty seemed to be feeling that she has become a burden for her daughter, due to her increased physical needs. The facilitator responded in a positive tone that did not seem to match Hetty's feelings.

> **Hetty:** I went to live with my, my daughter after I had the stroke, but it was a bit much for her, but, of it, I doubt it was in it. Nothing said or anything, but she had to take me to the toilet every, certain, day, mmm.
>
> **Facilitator:** She became your nurse, really, I suppose.
>
> **Hetty:** Yeah, yeah.
>
> **Facilitator:** Oh that was lovely.
>
> **Hetty:** I think she gets, get tired of taking me to the toilet.

The facilitator encouraged the group to think of special things about growing older, resulting in this exchange with Rose (in the same group as Hetty) in the excerpt below:

> **Facilitator:** Anyone else, just a comment, has someone got a comment, something good?
>
> **Rose:** I've lost my intelligence. I can't do things that I used to do. I seem a bit dumb to what I used to be. I do silly things, I do.
>
> **Facilitator:** I don't mean to laugh, I think it's lovely what you said.
>
> **Rose:** Yes I do, I said to J [daughter], 'I can't do what I used to do.' 'Well', she said, 'you are getting older'.

Session memos related to this session record a description of the quality of the relationship between the mother and daughter; it seems apparent that they were able to speak openly to each other.

Strategies for dealing with hard things

Sometimes with the depth of exchange in the group, humour is also seen, as in the exchange below. Humour was reported as a way into transcendence (MacKinlay 2006). The participant has an MMSE of only 13.

Interviewer: Is, you know, is your, does your faith help you in coping with the…

Anita: Oh yes.

Interviewer: Yeah.

Anita: Yes, I've er (*pause*) as I say I, I'm sort of working with them all but (*both laughs, missed words*) but you know.[4]

Interviewer: Yes.

Anita: And I, for to be strength, that is my prayer really.

Interviewer: Yeah.

Faith was also seen by some of the participants as providing strength for dealing with the hard things in life.

Interviewer: So what do you think it is that's helped you actually work through your issues of you know of loss and grief in a way that you've been able to cope?

Grace: My religion.

Interviewer: Yes.

Grace: Yes. It's a wonderful backup you know. It's just good.

Another of these participants, with an MMSE of 12, found faith a strong support and reported this as one of the good things:

Graham: Pardon me. The good things. Peace with God.

Interviewer: Yes.

Graham: Relationship with the Lord, holding onto that firm. That's another point of mine. Well if I can't expose anything or see it, and quite often I can't, I have got to, what pardon me, I have got to acknowledge a lot of the other things, and I have to care for Audrey, my wife, to see how she is going.

Summary

This chapter has focused on self-transcendence in ageing, and in particular in dementia. MacKinlay's (2006) model of the spiritual tasks and process of ageing identified transcendence as one of the important tasks of growing

---

4   In this and a few other exchanges, it may not be obvious to the reader what was funny, but it certainly caused both interviewer and participants to laugh. It may even be a form of connecting with people who have dementia.

older. Has the Enlightenment and modern society supported the growth of barriers against developing skills of transcendence? It appears that there is a tendency to want to abolish disability and dependency, rather than to find ways of transcending or overcoming. The need to struggle with difficulties in life is too often denied, opting to discard what no longer functions effectively in preference for a replacement. An old body, physical disabilities, mental disabilities, the desire is for cure or replacement; these desires do not lead to spiritual growth in later life, but rather to disappointment, despondency and despair.

How can people with dementia be encouraged to become more transcendent? One of the greatest barriers to increased transcendence is a lack of knowledge of what is possible. Ageism constricts and reinforces the stereotypes of ageing for those are growing older and society at large. Transcendence is possible for any older person, with or without dementia. Perhaps the person with dementia who has not developed some transcendence before the onset of their dementia may struggle more to come to a state of transcendence, perhaps not. We do not understand enough about this process to be certain.

In each of these chapters, it is worth remembering that the people whose words we have used and all the topics and concerns that they raise are similar to those we would expect of cognitively competent people too, yet these are people with dementia.

6

'You've Got to Laugh!'

A sense of humour is truly a human thing. As people age and become more physically and psychologically vulnerable and social networks become limited, humour may buffer the negative and enhance positive changes (Mak and Carpenter 2007). Humour emerged naturally among the participants in this study. In the spiritual reminiscence groups there was much laughter as participants laughed at themselves and their situation or recalled amusing past events. Again as we listened to the laughter in groups it was easy to forget that each participant had dementia. Kimble claims that humour may express a 'heroic defiance in the face of life's most crushing and challenging experiences' (Kimble 2004, p.7). Humour is seen to be very important in facing life's adversities. The ability to see humour in even the most dire events is viewed as an important coping mechanism. This can occur by offering a different way of viewing the adversity – and perhaps leading to laughter which can help to overcome feelings of depression, anxiety or anger (Martin 2009). Frankl (1984) noted that being able to overcome adversity through humour is one of the 'soul's weapons in the fight for self-preservation' (p.63). Humour is a part of most everyday interactions. This can be in the form of banter, teasing irony or joke telling. In this chapter we will discuss the underlying importance of humour and laughter for older people and then talk about some specific examples of humour noted in the small groups.

Humour across the centuries

The term humour is derived from the Latin word *humor* meaning moisture. This moisture refers to the four body fluids – blood, phlegm, black bile and yellow bile. The relative amounts of each of these fluids influenced a person's physical and personal disposition. Over time it came to refer to the dispositions themselves and finally to the character of the person (Oring 2010). There have been many approaches to defining humour over time.

The Greeks two and a half millennia ago were fascinated by the concept of laughter and what it meant. Since then, questions have continued to be asked about humour: Why do we laugh? What do we laugh at? and What are the consequences of that laughter? (Oring 2010, p.*ix*).

Over the centuries various philosophers and psychologists have theorised about the role and definition of humour. In the 16th century Hobbes proposed the 'Superiority Theory or Tendentious or Disparagement Theory'. This was considered an aggressive form of humour which takes pleasure in others' failings or discomfort (McCreaddie and Wiggins 2008). If we look back to our recent times – possibly as recently as the 1960s – we will certainly see examples of this type of humour. In our own lifetime we have seen a change in the type of humour that we feel comfortable using. It is certainly regarded as 'politically incorrect' to make fun of or laugh at those who are less fortunate or have other physical or mental deformities. It is possibly even more disturbing to note that for the last 400 years it has been acceptable to joke about these matters!

In the 18th century the philosopher Kant (1724–1804) proposed the Incongruity Theory – the punch-line or resolution is incongruent with the set-up (McCreaddie and Wiggins 2008). In this category we can identify jokes that, during the 20th century until now, have become the mainstay of comedy shows of one kind or another. Because recognising the incongruity in jokes is a complex mental task, there have been a number of studies on the older person's capacity to understand jokes as a measure of humour appreciation and cognitive ability. There are even tools to measure humour such as the Joke and Story Completion Test. This test is widely used in humour research and is a measure based on the incongruity–resolution theory of humour (Brownell *et al.* 1983 cited in Mak and Carpenter 2007). It is also important to be aware that humour is culturally defined and may thus differ between different cultural groups.

In the 20th century Freud (1856–1939) proposed that humour was released by 'excess' nervous energy, which actually masks other motives and desires. He referred to this as 'Relief or Release Theory' (McCreaddie and Wiggins 2008). In humour and jokes, some aggressive and sexual impulses can be made more socially acceptable (Oring 2010). This can again be seen in many comedy shows – and the jokes made in the pub or clubhouse; many of these certainly are not 'politically correct'! It does also indicate how humour can relieve tension in a difficult situation.

The definition generally accepted now is that humour is an amusing communication consisting of multiple incongruous meanings (Martin 2007).

However, McFadden (2004) notes that humour 'resists neat definitions' (p.17). Humour consists of many subcategories, and the many books written on humour frequently disagree on how to define these subcategories (McFadden 2004). Humour can occur in many everyday situations and can be divided into three broad categories: jokes (humorous anecdotes that are passed on); spontaneous humour that occurs in social situations; and accidental or unintended humour (Martin 2007). Humour involves both cognitive and emotional elements. Humour is a pleasurable experience. Exposure to humour can cause an increase in positive affect and mood (Szabo 2003 cited in Martin 2007). When using ethnography, by means of observations of people with dementia in aged care facilities over several months, McFadden, Ingram and Baldauf (2000) found that these people used humour in everyday situations, where most humour involved 'banal' situations, and not in response to pre-prepared jokes. They related this to Frankl's work on humour, noting that they had mastered 'the art of living'. McFadden *et al.* (2000) commented that these people demonstrated a triumph of the human spirit as they continued living with a progressive and debilitating disease, still finding humour in everyday living.

Although we often think about laughter as indicating a humorous or happy situation, it is also evident in times of relief, hysteria, nervousness and horror (Oring 2010). When listening to the transcripts, however, it was evident that most of the laughter was in response to a humorous interaction initiated by the group members themselves. Laughter is reputed to provide a number of additional physiological benefits. Berk (2010) has summarised a number of these including improving respiration and circulation; decreasing stress hormones; increasing the levels of endorphins; and improving mental functioning. He proposes that 'laughter does offer sedentary elderly folk an alternative' and suggests that adding laughter to an exercise programme or even replacing the exercise programme with laughter is a definite advantage (p.332). Kitwood (1993) has identified humour as one of his 12 indicators of personal well-being in moderate or severe dementia. Social interactions of those with dementia are often significantly limited – the sharing of laughter can help to enhance the bonds between those with dementia and their family and community. Personal narratives introduce fun into an interaction and offer a way for others to participate (Norrick 2009). The presence of humour shows that the human spirit has not been vanquished – there is still hope (Kimble 2004).

Humour, however, can also be harmful to psychological well-being. Self-defeating humour can be harmful to one's self-esteem. Self-defeating humour includes making jokes about oneself or allowing others to make the person the 'butt' of the jokes, ostensibly to gain acceptance from others (Martin 2009). Hostile humour is intentionally mean-spirited. In hostile humour there is no attempt to make the person happy – rather it is used to undermine, humiliate and ridicule. Hostile or aggressive humour inflicts injury, 'either to self or to one's relationship with others', without concern for its harmful impact on others. Belittling others is an example of this form of humour (Martin 2009). This is making humour at the expense of others. Much ageist humour takes this perspective and can be very demeaning to older people. Martin (2009) believes that this negative type of humour can perhaps be deleterious to well-being. When studying humour, it is important to also identify the type of humour that is being used. Older adults, however, compared with younger adults, were less likely to use aggressive forms of humour or use humour to disparage or control others (Martin *et al.* 2003).

MacKinlay (2004, 2006) found that humour could provide a way into transcendence among older cognitively competent people. She noted that older people often make jokes about memory loss and would tend to identify it with growing older, rather than with dementia. Using her model of the spiritual tasks of ageing, it is possible to see how this process of self-transcendence can be promoted through humour, and also that humour may occur more frequently when the person has gained some sense of peace and comfort in their life. Of course, personality may also be a factor in humour, and provides another variable between humour as expressed and appreciated by others. Authentic humour may well be a sign of a degree of transcendence. Thus humour is more likely to occur when the person feels sure of their identity and has developed some spiritual maturity (McFadden 2004). To what degree can people with dementia continue to engage with the use of humour? MacKinlay's model of the spiritual tasks and process of ageing shows linkages between humour and transcendence (see Figure 6.1).

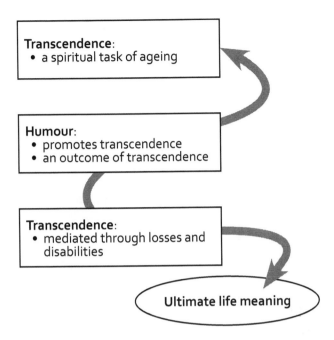

Figure 6.1 *Self-transcendence and humour: A spiritual process related to life-meaning (from MacKinlay 2006)*

Expressions of humour by people with dementia in the spiritual reminiscence groups

Humour and laughter reinforce the sense of identity. Older people with dementia tend to lose their identity – they become the person with dementia rather than themselves. In the groups there was the opportunity to establish new relationships and share stories – each of these helped to support identity. The following excerpt is from the observational journal kept by the research assistant. The facilitator here encourages the interactions and helps Hetty to join in and contribute. Through reminding her about family photos, she is able to trigger those additional memories. As the research assistant notes, Rose is enjoying the attention that she has received as part of the group.

> Hetty talks again about parties: likes family parties. Says she hasn't got a big family.
> The facilitator says: what about all those photos in your room?
> Hetty says they're my family. She laughed at being caught out, and others laughed with her.

Rose used to have a full social life. She made the group laugh at her stories. She appeared to be pleased with the group's attention.

Both these interactions highlight how humour is used among group members. In a study about humour in community-dwelling older people, it was found that participants grounded their references to humour in contexts that were shared with others – family members and friends. Humour was an essential part of forming a positive outlook on life and maintaining social connections. Having a sense of humour was valued and seen as essential to manage the losses of function that accompany the ageing process (Damianakis and Marziali 2011). In the following excerpt Rose makes the group laugh with her humour:

Facilitator: What's the best part of the day, Rose?

Rose: After dinner. I have fallen, after ten minutes I am off to sleep, and I wake up when it's tea-time. (*everyone laughs*)

The following discussion arose from a question about reading the Bible. This example shows a great deal of humour and genuine fun – and identifies how despite older age and dementia, a strong sense of humour prevails. This is also quite a complex interaction between two participants – the facilitator joins in later in the interaction but has not done anything to keep the conversation going.

Ruby: But to me the Bible is very sombre book – don't hear anyone smiling or laughing do you in the Bible – not at all.

Bob: Well, why should it be – I wonder do they laugh when they're not writing Bible stories?

Ruby: I like to hear some fun – very sombre.

Bob: It is – very serious.

Ruby: Yes.

Bob: There's no light-heartedness in it at all – it's all serious.

Facilitator: It's serious, you're saying.

Bob: Yes, very serious…

Facilitator: You don't think it's serious or not – joking funny laughing.

Bob: I think being about God it would have to be – well, it wouldn't have to be serious – no but they made it like that – they haven't recorded any of their happiest days – they're all dismal – you can see them all with long faces like the pictures of them. Can't you, Ruby?

Ruby: Yes, and I think it's something that happened in those days perhaps.

Bob: I'm not sure – they must have had a laugh and a giggle I think – oh, they'd have to – but they haven't recorded any of that, no, it's all…

It is also good to see how the group picks up on the humour the facilitator uses.

Facilitator: What are you looking forward to, Louise?

Louise: Oh, I am too tired. (*laughs*) Time to get things, right, really.

Facilitator: I hope that we will finish this discussion. (*everyone laughs*)

Humour as a coping strategy and a means to spiritual self-transcendence

Using humour can help older people reframe past events. Even those events surrounding the death of loved ones can be reframed by focusing on almost prosaic events that happened in connection with the painful events. Humorous stories are an effective strategy for thinking through negative life events that are intrinsic to being a great age (Matsumoto 2009). We found this ourselves in the groups. Many times that laughter was evident in the groups was when participants were talking about either potentially sad events such as their own death, or past sad events. In a study of hospice care it was found that humour was present in over 85 per cent of all nurse visits, whether the person was in a hospice, nursing home or in their own home. The only time when there was not a humorous interaction was when the person was in the final stages of dying and unable to contribute to the conversations. Dying patients initiated more episodes of humour than their family, carers or nurses (Adamle and Ludwick 2005). Combined with caring and sensitivity, humour proved to be a powerful therapeutic asset in hospice/palliative care.

In the following excerpt we can see how the theme of life and death is discussed with some humour. One of the participants – aged 97 – was frequently bemoaning the fact that she did not have long to live. This became a repeated theme during the 24-week group.[1]

Freda: See, I haven't got long to live.

Mavis: Oh, here we go again!

Facilitator: It was bound to come up, wasn't it?

1 The excerpt is from the pilot study conducted prior to the main study and therefore these participants are not listed in Appendix 2.

June: Look, tell us when to wring the handkerchiefs.

Freda: No…you've err three years to live.

June: Who told you that?

Facilitator: Is that just because you'll be 100 in three years? That doesn't mean that's when you have to finish, you can go on to be 110.

Mavis: That, you'll be here to annoy us.

Facilitator: That's right. And we'll all be saying, when you're 105 – I thought you said you were going when you were 100.

The following is an example of ironical humour in response to a question about feelings of growing older:

Facilitator: How do you feel about growing older?

June: It becomes a habit.

Summary

The use of humour was evident in all the groups – no matter what the discussion was about. It helped to reinforce the companionship experienced in the groups and enhance individuals' sense of identity. When facilitating spiritual reminiscence groups the facilitator needs to be aware of interpreting and managing humour that is damaging or self-defeatist and to help support the group.

7

Wisdom and Insight

There are many ways of looking at wisdom. However, we often assume that the 'wise' person is not frequently encountered, is probably elderly and perhaps somewhat remote, perhaps some kind of a guru. First, it may be hard to imagine wisdom among ordinary older people, as Kenyon *et al.* (2001) have suggested, or second, to imagine wisdom among people who have dementia, if the normally accepted paradigms are the basis for knowledge of the characteristics of people with dementia. However, in the transcripts of these small groups and in-depth interviews, wisdom of a spiritual nature is demonstrated. In the context of this study, wisdom has to do with the ability to live with ambiguity and uncertainty and to be at peace.

Wisdom in ageing

Erikson's well-known stages of psychosocial development across the life-span have the eighth stage as negotiating integrity versus despair and, as an outcome, wisdom. It is too much to claim a complete sense of integrity or of despair in any instance, but the move would likely be towards one or the other side of the continuum. As Erikson wrote (Erikson *et al.* 1986), it was in this final stage of struggle between integrity and despair that it was also possible for the psychosocial stages to weave back on one another, as the person may reflect and grapple with earlier stages of development, noting the possibility of a spiralling nature of development. In 1997, Erikson's widow, Joan, completed a further edition of the book *The Life Cycle Completed*. She included a ninth stage of development, acknowledging the effects of increasing frailty in extreme old age, of the late eighties and nineties. Examination of the stages of psychosocial development in later life drew MacKinlay to consider a spiritual dimension to this eighth stage, and a spiritual perspective of wisdom. She defined a spiritual concept of wisdom in later life as:

> An increased tolerance to uncertainty, a deepening search for meaning in life, including an awareness of the paradoxical and contradictory nature of reality; it involves transcendence of uncertainty and a move from external to internal regulation. (MacKinlay 2001a, p.153)

This definition is given in contrast to definitions of wisdom that often focus on cognitive function, including intelligence and memory as the basis of conferring wisdom on the particular person. The position taken in this book is on the grappling with ambiguities and uncertainties of later life, especially during the later periods of frailty and disabilities. It is argued that people may still exhibit wisdom, even when they may have some degree of cognitive impairment. Frail older people can show wisdom; we believe that people with dementia can also show evidence of wisdom, defined as it is in this chapter.

Wisdom in a spiritual context

Although a lot of research has been conducted into a psychological perspective of wisdom (Sternberg 1990), this has mainly focused on psychological constructs of wisdom. A spiritual view of wisdom is needed to explain the complexity and possibilities of later life development that includes successful ageing, frailty and mental health. The field of narrative gerontology offers new insights into wisdom and the spiritual perspective in later life. Randall and Kenyon (2004) offer a way of understanding wisdom in ageing, along with its relationship with the spiritual dimension:

> …when aging is considered as a biographical process, in which, over time, we are continually storying or composing (Bateson, 1993) our lives, then we are permitted a fresh perspective on the spiritual dimension of the developmental process. Integral to that dimension, we submit, is the unique wisdom to which our stories afford us access. (Randall and Kenyon 2004, p.335)

We see this narrative approach to wisdom as a valuable way of engaging with life-meaning for older adults, and not least with those who have dementia. This is the approach of Randall and Kenyon (2004), which acknowledges not the 'what' of wisdom so much as the 'how' of wisdom that is of importance. In other words, it is the meaning of the life story that is important; in contrast, the facts of the life story are of lesser consequence. That is, whatever wisdom is understood to be – enlightenment, good judgement, compassion, union with God – it comes alive only in our unique wisdom stories. When it comes to wisdom, what may seem an inconsequential or ordinary insight to one person may be a truly extraordinary insight for another (Randall and Kenyon 2004).

Hence, we may ask, how do people see meaning in life? Randall and Kenyon see story telling, the listening to story and meditation upon it as all being important for the growing of wisdom in later life. They write of 'storying moments' and suggest that these can be facilitated in various ways. It is actually within this context that we have approached our work in spiritual reminiscence for people with dementia. Until this point, there seems to have been nothing published in the area of wisdom, spirituality, ageing and dementia. It seems that there is the potential for real value for these people to engage with their life-meaning in the present, drawing on what they remember as meaningful from their past. This will allow a sense of acceptance and perhaps peace as they face a future of uncertainty and ambiguity, which we all face; it is only that people with dementia may be more aware of this than are people who are 'cognitively competent'.

> Each instant, we are presented with an enormous cognitive dilemma. Technically, the present is all there is; yet it is perpetually receding from reach, only to be replaced by another present, which in turn is all there is. To manoeuvre from one fleeting instant of presentness to the next, we form images of previous instants, more or less connected, to give ourselves some sense of substance, a sense we experience as 'the past'. Thus, by *imag-ination*, we make the past present again. We re-present it. These re-presentations, however, are not exact replicas of what occurred, but 'texts' that we weave from the bare events and objective circumstances of our raw existence. (Randall and Kenyon 2004, p.334)

Randall and Kenyon write that the three time modes of past, present and future continually modify each other, and that this intermingling of the modes is 'so integral to our lives that most of the time we are unconscious of its occurrence' (Randall and Kenyon 2004, p.334). They note the importance of differentiating between clock time and human time that is narrative time or story time. Further, Randall and Kenyon draw on the writings of Ray to explain how wisdom features in the reimagining of story in later life. Ray's work was with older women: 'Wise people,' Ray writes, 'watch themselves tell life stories, learn from others' stories, and intervene in their own narrative processes to allow for change by admitting new stories and interpretations into their repertoire' (Ray quoted in Randall and Kenyon 2004, p.339). This account is of value in seeing how reminiscence may work in later life, to assist the person to come to a sense of their final life-meaning, and a sense of peace and acceptance through re-storying and reimagining of the meaning of one's individual life story or narrative. This work was done with cognitively competent older adults. Could a similar process work for people with dementia? Are people with dementia able to reimagine? Are people with dementia aware enough to draw on relevant aspects of their past to reminisce adequately in the present to enable a coming to meaning? Can they see themselves in this process of growing and becoming?

Wisdom among people with dementia

One question that can be asked of people with dementia is whether, as their cognition declines, they can retain wisdom, or second, whether they can continue to develop wisdom, perhaps not related to cognitive function, as in intelligence, but perhaps exhibiting wisdom of a spiritual nature. If so, might this be a wisdom that enables them to come to a sense of peace and joy, even in the midst of dementia, and the losses that it brings? How do we see signs of wisdom in a person? It seems that in a spiritual perspective we would look for signs of integrity, peace and joy. We might also see if the person shows any signs of insight into their situation or the situations of others. It is in this way that we have examined the transcripts of in-depth interviews and the group sessions to find examples of wisdom.

What does a spiritual view of wisdom look like?

From the foregoing discussion it seems that a spiritual view of wisdom would be seen through evidence of signs of self-awareness, being able to live with uncertainty and ambiguity, and evidence of peace and joy. The opposite of this would be signs of anxiety, distress and despair. These people may also show signs of courage as they face their uncertain future. This construct is not an absolute one; rather it is a continuum. Thus at one extreme the person would show signs of anxiety and despair, while at the other there would be signs of peace and joy.

Wisdom – examples of insight from the study

We tapped into the spiritual aspect of wisdom through questions that led to final meanings. This assumed some processing of the meaning of life, grappling with difficult things, rejoicing in blessings and finding a sense of peace in acceptance of life experiences. Obviously wisdom has to do with insight, and this is supposed by many to be lacking in dementia. The following questions formed the overall framework for this section:

- What gives greatest meaning to your life now? *And follow up with questions like:*
  - What is most important in your life?
  - What keeps you going?
  - Is life worth living? Why is life worth living?
- Looking back over your life:
  - What do you remember with joy?
  - What do you remember with sadness?

Questions that elicited responses related to wisdom were situated around joy, sadness, hope, what it was like growing older, hard things in life, life-meaning and fears. These were often asked within the themes of the model of the spiritual tasks of ageing. We examined the transcripts of both in-depth interviews and small group sessions to find examples that would fit with this major theme.

Joy and sadness

First we have looked at instances of responses to questions on joy. Joy could be seen as a sign of integrity and wisdom as we have defined it in this chapter. We would wish to distinguish between happiness and joy. Happiness seems a more superficial emotion than joy. Happiness assumes a 'feel good', 'happy', all is right with the world impression. On the other hand, joy plumbs the very depths of what it means to be human. Joy can be present even in the presence of pain. It is an assurance of goodness and integrity, even in the face of suffering. We did not specifically ask questions about happiness, but only joy. However, we did include questions on sadness to address the continuum of that emotion. We received mixed responses, as would be expected because of the individual life stories; the examples below are indicative of the range received.

Pausing to consider before answering, this participant, Jill (MMSE 3), responded initially to the question of joy by simply stating 'I'm a mother' and then unpacking what that meant to her. This seemed to be part of her story, a part of her identity, of being a mother, but also being a teacher. Obviously it has been necessary to make inferences from the words of these people. The reader may like to reflect on what these examples show about people with dementia and their ability to negotiate abstract and deep aspects of life, while perhaps finding it difficult to find the most appropriate words to express themselves.

Interviewer: Yes, before I came in, yes. When you look back over your life, what things do you remember as times of joy? What times, times of joy? What things were really special things that brought you joy in life?

Jill: I'm a mother.

Interviewer: Yes. That says a lot.

Jill: Well it is a lot.

Interviewer: Yes, indeed.

Jill: I would say, and you have got to have a home clean and tidy, and being a mother you've got to have food and lots of things. Be good manager for a start, especially if you have got to go to work to help, look after your families, if you have a family.

Interviewer: And did you have to go to work then, when you had your family?

Jill: No, when I had a family, I went much more, much more tired at night, because I was always teaching, and that's not correct, be a good tired person like, for instance, if your school teacher was a bit rough, did not have time to do it, you would not like them, would you?

Interviewer: No.

Jill: Well that's the same with your work.

Interviewer: That's right.

Jill: But the only difference is, at work, I would say, be more careful how you spoke to people, depending on of course what work you wanted, and be accepted, I would say, but if you are accepted, you accept these people in work, they mightn't think the job is done properly, so you ask them to speak (*pause*) that is not a very nice thing to say, or something like that. You will try a bit more, because it is earning you money. So that's about all I can say.

This same woman then responded to the question of sadness. It is interesting that she expressed her need to reflect on this question before she could respond. She then showed by her response, where some words seem to be mixed, her understanding of wisdom:

Interviewer: Looking back over your life, we just talked about things to do with joy, what things would you remember that were sad things in your life?

Jill: Well I am going to try to say those sort of things, no I would have to take, a little bit to think about it. You would not, if you would have to say that part in your life, you would not try to *be* nice, you have to be naturally those sorts of things.

Interviewer: You are speaking a lot of wisdom here. That's wisdom, what you are saying.

Jill: Is it?

Interviewer: Yes.

Jill: Oh, tick him off.

Interviewer: Tick it off, oh that's good.

Jill: No well, if you were interested in it really, you would do it naturally, wouldn't you?

Interviewer: Yes of course you would, yes, that's right.

Jill: Would not matter what subject I had to do, this is only me.

Interviewer: Well that's what we are interested in, is you.

Jill: Well I would say hmm, if somebody came up to talk to me, and I did not quite like how they spoke, or when they interrupted if they knew you were talking or whatever like that, I would try and draw it out first, to see what they are like. I don't know if that is the right thing to do.

The importance of family was spoken of. Note too that this question also brought out responses of sorrow, not joy, and it is assumed that this type of response was elicited because the question also drew out the negative emotions of the same theme – what was in the person's mind, not only the specific emotion of 'joy' that was asked about. We have found that study participants would respond to the question in a much broader way, in that they would seem to take in the actual question of 'joy' and find that what they had to speak of was sorrow, and so they responded from this perspective.

Was it that they didn't understand? We don't think that was the case; rather, they interpreted the question to mean the spectrum of that emotion which could also encompass sorrow and suffering as well as joy. Is this a sign that these people were able to respond more deeply to emotions than it might be assumed? What cognitive processing was going on here that produced these answers?

Were some of these answers actually evidence of wisdom amongst these vulnerable people? We would like to suggest that they are. Of course, suggesting this raises further questions about brain function and processing of emotions, which goes beyond the cognitive.

Facilitator: Yes (*pause*) it's very important. (*pause*) When you look back over your life what, what would be the things that you remember with most joy?

Amy: Well I suppose to most women who've had a family um, when your children are born you know, there's nothing that can be greater, greater, bring greater joy than that, and er (*pause*) of course er well we've had um, in my life time I've seen, well, I was born at the end of the 1914–18 war.

Facilitator: Yes, right, now what else? When you look back over your life, what are the things that bring you most joy?

Anita: (*pause*) Joy? Mmm (*long pause*) er (*long pause*) I know I, I was quite young but I was suffering from, from lack of care.

Facilitator: Mmm.

Anita: And er, though I had wonderful parents mind you, but er (*pause*) er and er one of my sisters got in touch with my father who I'm afraid had broken the marriage, which never should have happened, because it was always a very good marriage.

Facilitator: So what would you say have been the high points, the really joyful times in your life?

Grace: Well, marriage.

Facilitator: Yes, yes, now I wonder if you could perhaps share with me some of the high spots or some of the times in your life that have been particularly filled with joy.

Jane: I can't think of any, anything that, I think Christmas always brings me a lot of joy.

Facilitator: Right, yes.

Jane: I enjoy Christmas. We usually go out together, the whole family, and it brings a lot of joy and you see people you haven't seen for awhile and that's always good.

As suggested above, the question of joy sometimes also brought memories of sadness, as in the excerpt from the in-depth interview below:

Interviewer: That's good. When you look back over your life, what are the things you remember as special times of joy?

Rose: Oh, I was very joyful in life, very happy, I thought… (*trails off*)

Interviewer: Yes you were happy then.

Rose: I was a very happy girl. My friends have all gone. (*crying*)

Interviewer: Yep, so what were the high points, the things that you remember particularly, the happy times?

Rose: Well I used to go out, my husband died, buried him, when I went out with another fellow that also lost his wife, don't know what it's called, we were in a Saxon home, and I had to not stay flat for a while, I had my home, and it's cleaning, and I thought, I used to pay a lady to come once a week and clean around for me, and then my friend, was husband's, and my friend, I remember I used to go up to a club every Friday, Saturday, I had a nice time, but now everything is gone.

Interviewer: So there has been a lot of things, a lot of losses you have had in recent times. That's very sad. So.

Rose: So my daughter brought me over from England to be with her for...

Interviewer: Had you ever lived in Australia before?

Rose: No, I used to come over for holidays.

Interviewer: For holidays, yes.

Rose: And I was quite happy then because my husband used to come with me.

Interviewer: Yes, and that's different, isn't it?

Rose: Yes, well the last time we came out here together, we used to come out here for three months at a time.

Interviewer: Yes.

Rose: For three months, was about October, was about the time we went back, and he, we went back home Sunday, we went back home I think Saturday or Sunday, and in the next Sunday he went out to the lavatory, and he fell in, collapsed and died, straight away. He was gone.

Interviewer: Just so suddenly. That must have been a great shock to you.

Rose: He was only 68.

Interviewer: That's quite young, isn't it?

Rose: Hmmm. He always had, he never said he had a bad heart, but you would always wonder about it, but he would not have anything to do with doctors, or go to the doctors, no it's alright (*pause*) and so he's gone.

Interviewer: Yes, and just suddenly you were alone?

Rose: Yes.

The following narrative is from a woman who was a member of a fundamentalist religious group when she was younger. It shows her struggle and the ways that she has attempted to reconcile her beliefs and her losses through her journey. Again, the story that emerged was of sadness when the interviewer asked about the experiences of joy:

> **Interviewer:** I want to ask you now, looking back over your life for a little while, what are the things that you remember with joy, as you look back over your life?
>
> **Daphne:** Not very much.
>
> **Interviewer:** Not very much. So there, no special times that you, in your life.
>
> **Daphne:** Not really, because, I don't know whether you know the Brethren?
>
> **Interviewer:** I know about them.
>
> **Daphne:** Some are called exclusive, there are all kinds of Brethrens, open Brethrens, they are very good. The exclusive Brethren, with whom I was brought up, and lived my first 20 years, uh, and although a lot of their beliefs don't conform with the majority of ideas, uh, in that they seem harsh, and cruel, I do know that that is their belief and I was brought up to believe that was so, so I don't condemn them in any way, I don't belong to them just now.

Daphne described a very sad life, with the loss of a child and an unhappy marriage, outside of her religious beliefs. She then went on to say:

> **Daphne:** But that's the start. I have got a story, but it is all sad.
>
> **Interviewer:** It's sad?
>
> **Daphne:** And when you say what's happy, it isn't.
>
> **Interviewer:** Well I wanted to ask you both sides, I wanted to ask you what were the things you remembered with joyful things, and then I was going to ask you.
>
> **Daphne:** One of the joyful things is when, I have been to the service this morning, and that is my biggest joy, very biggest spiritual uplift. You caught me on a good day, because I was spiritually uplifted at the moment.
>
> **Interviewer:** That's wonderful.

As Daphne reflected in the process of telling her story, she showed insight into her life values and beliefs, differentiating between the facts of her life story and the way that one can overcome adversity through changing attitudes. The interview went on to conclude:

> **Daphne:** Everything that has happened, happened. Nobody can change it, and it's just God has given me different things to think about.
>
> **Interviewer:** Yes.
>
> **Daphne:** But that's all sorts of things have gone, gone out. Um, after the war, before we sold everything up and things, L, my husband, came back, we had another child, it lived ten days, another one gone.
>
> **Interviewer:** That is so sad.
>
> **Daphne:** That's, no it's more than that. Never mind, I can smile, I (*pause*)…

Overcoming and living within restrictions

In this in-depth interview Don speaks of his difficulties with the rules of the care facility that he now resides in; he shares his experiences of failing health and associated disability. He begins by speaking of his difficulty in dealing with putting any goals into practice and coping with a real loss of independence. Yet, it seems there is wisdom here in his reflections of the situation that he finds himself in, even if he cannot work through how do achieve the independence he wants:

> **Don:** The most important thing I worry about is lack of, uh, my own intention to do anything.
>
> **Interviewer:** Mmm hmm.
>
> **Don:** Because when you are in a place like this, you just have to carry out the rules and regulations, and allow things to take their course.
>
> **Interviewer:** Mmm.
>
> **Don:** Whereas when if I was on my own as I was for some time before I came in here, I could go and come as I liked. I could eat or not eat as I liked.
>
> **Interviewer:** Mmm.
>
> **Don:** And in that way my initiative was not undermined.
>
> **Interviewer:** Mmm, mmm.

Don: But there is no such thing as initiative here. It is all rules and regulations. And if you try to be insistent, you upset the whole system, and that doesn't do anybody any good. And uh, and I have had one or two bad spells of health, which has, uh, knocked me down quite a lot. In fact I am just recovering from a bit of pneumonia.

Interviewer: Mmm.

Don: But thank goodness it is passing away.

Interviewer: It is settled.

Don: So, that is one of the things which was telling on me really much when I first came in here.

Interviewer: Mmm.

Don: But by the help of people of the church, particularly who came around to see me, and knew me from the days that I was able to... Also the biggest problem I have is that my sight failed.

Interviewer: Oh, okay.

Don: And as a result of that, I am almost totally blind, and that prevents me from doing anything at all. However good, bad or otherwise on my own initiative. I have lost that initiative as a result of that. And everything that I do is more or less governed by that disability.

Interviewer: Mmm.

Don: And even now I will never recognise you again, except if I spoke to you.

Interviewer: Yeah, yeah.

Don: Because I can't see you.

Interviewer: You can't see me.

Don: But uh, sometimes, my vision is such, for instance I can see that you are wearing a green top and dark pants.

Interviewer: Mmm mmm.

Don: So that much, at close range, I can see now. If you just walked away I would not see that at all.

Interviewer: Mmm. Can you read?

Don: No.

Interviewer: Mmm.

Don: So I have to depend very heavily on my old radio.

Interviewer: So you…

Don: And people come and read to me of course and so on.

Interviewer: And I was going to say, what are the hardest things in your life just now? Would that be losing your sight?

Don: That is the biggest, yes.

Loss of memory and sense of identity

June (MMSE 6) struggled with her sense of identity with the crucial words: 'I can't, don't remember who I am and what I am and what, what, who.' Her memory and identity problems were obviously on her mind, as she returned to the topic later in the same interview (see below), speaking of her speech problems. June seemed to have insight into the fact of her memory and speech problems, and she could share that in the one-on-one interview. Part of wisdom, in a spiritual perspective, is the ability to live with uncertainty and ambiguity; it appears that this was certainly the case here.

June: A couple of English girls that have been there for a long time. Were there for a long time, I think it was, they must had both their husbands were tired or something, and they have been there, and yes, they stay calm. But the last thing I think is that even then, when I'm, people, I can't, don't remember who I am and what I am and what, what, who.

Interviewer: Do you find that hard?

June: The right back, not that way, I know all the backers, you know, it's the things that have come, this own time, you know, but I just can't just stick. I can't do things at times now, I can't do that.

Later in the same interview June returned to the subject:

Interviewer: Do you take part in anything now? Any of the activities here, these are church services or the Bible readings, all the prayer meetings.

June: No, not at the moment.

Interviewer: Not at the moment.

June: No, I just sort of feel as if I don't at the moment, uh, because I just sort of been loved, and uh, feeling to, um, mmm. And I just don't see, now it's very difficult.

Interviewer: Getting more difficult?

June: Well that's right, because you just don't keep people. I mean I go to say something, and it does not go out.

Interviewer: You get a little bit jumbly with words do you?

June: Oh God, terrible.

There was more to June than simply concerns about a loss of identity. She could respond to the broad questions, even if not specifically; mixing and confusion of words was obvious, but she was able to respond in the general topic area. We have included a long excerpt from her transcript here to follow through on her thought processes; looking carefully, it can be seen that she is responding to the questions that were asked:

Interviewer: Do you have an image of a God at all?

June: Well, well I don't know about that. But yes, but I mean we were always at school, the girls and me, and were there, and so forth, until later on, long time when you get up and you think, and you think now, you are busy and you don't do it. Yes. We all went to church, but then, when they were small, when they went, had, had their everything, and we did, didn't I used to look after them, and Ron, my husband, used to, when they have to work, on Sunday, for Sunday, can't, I was Monday. He would be home, and have some time, and he'd be, go out there helping build the men, to build up an extra church with a bit something.

Interviewer: Oh okay.

June: He was, it sounds too so silly, but that was my husband was very much like that. Could do for and told for. Talks. You could hear him from here, from here to, but everybody loved him.

Interviewer: A good talker was he?

June: Yes, that's right. And uh, they always loved him, and every, all the kids used to like him, and things, and he'll just, he would always find someone when we would be going on a holiday in the cars, and he always stopped, and looked to see what Mr J, my friend, stopped, he does not look as if he has got it on the right place. (*laughs*) You know and it was just, but all said just was the way the life was. Christian. Loved him, bigger than me.

Interviewer: And um, do you see that your, how do you see your spiritual needs being met now?

June: Well I don't think I can feel it.

Interviewer: Mmm hmm.

June: I mean I know, I hope I would go to God, but if I have not, it's because I have not done the right thing. But yes, I, I just feel, um, I suppose it's not a hard thing for you, because I have been like I am now,

I am not the girl that you could get out of, if you have gone that. But I was always, altogether, I was doing the, all the things, we always.

Louise, with an MMSE of just four, was having considerable difficulties communicating, and the following is from her in-depth interview transcript; note the interviewer asked how old she was, and this was a question Louise was not able to answer:

Interviewer: Uh huh. What would you say are the hardest things for you now?

Louise: Oh I don't know really, I am here, here.

Interviewer: Oh, it is hard to fix it. It's hard to get the words in?

Louise: Yes, it's, yes. I can't mix things up really.

Interviewer: Yes, yes, that happens sometimes.

Louise: Yes. Well it has been a long time, no wonder I have. (*laughs*)

Interviewer: How old are you now?

Louise: How old? Oh dear.

Interviewer: That's another hard one.

Louise: Oh yes (*laughs*) yes.

The following excerpts on the theme of joy were typical of responses. A simple memory of joy is summed up by this woman:

Interviewer: Yes, and as you look back over your life now, what are the things that you would see as being, the things you remember with joy?

Catherine: Being with my husband and enjoying everything with him.

Yet another woman had so much joy in her life:

Interviewer: So err looking back on your life now, what are the things you remember with a sense of joy?

Bronwyn: Oh. Oh there's so many, I couldn't.

Interviewer: Hmm.

Bronwyn: My daughter coming through her nursing career, and err I just don't know.

Yet another story included memories of migrating from England and life in the Australian bush:

Interviewer: So when you look back on your life now, what do you remember as times of joy?

John: Well let me go back. I was born in England in 1918, and we came out to Australia in 1925. And I was err eight, and I'll always remember it because, you may have already heard this story, because I don't ever remember seeing a dog, I'd seen horses in London, but nothing else. And err in October we arrived in Australia 1925 and we got off the ship, this is a real thing with me. We got off the ship and err in Sydney Harbour on a Friday, and on the Friday evening I had already travelled by train to Gosford, got in the T model Ford truck and travelled 22 miles to the bush, on an orchard, and err with Mum and Dad. And on the Monday I went to school, I walked three mile to school in bare feet.

Interviewer: Wow.

John: And err we went to school in a one-room classroom with a sixth level of education. And err I thought it was a wonderful start, because not only it was a school, but also my uncle being a bushman, he said, 'Right-oh Brownie you're old enough to carry a little rifle.' So I used to go out with them Uncle and Dad with guns and that, I had my rifle and shoot rabbits. Then of course within two years we were down in the city, because the depression started and there wasn't enough to keep all the families going on the farm. And of course being the depression I never went to school, bare feet, a patch across your trousers and that. And that's how I schooled; I was very active in various different things. We were a hardy mob I suppose in those days. But we, but then in 1932 I left school, because we had to because of the depression. And from then on I did a course and the war came in and I joined up and I was gone for six years. And since then of course I've been active in different things, and managed to have a job all the time. And we've had reasonably good health, and we went from house to house in those days with the rations, and when I came home um we bought a house. From then on you know it's been a peg, but we got over it.

Another example of sadness overwhelming any sense of joy in life can be seen in Sophie's interview:

Interviewer: Oh no, okay, um, other special times in your life, what other special things do you remember, things that perhaps were joyful times in your life?

Sophie: Joyful?

Interviewer: Yes.

Sophie: Or because the thing that comes to mind is that my only brother died when we was ah I think it was about ten year old.

Interviewer: Yes.

Sophie: He had leukaemia.

Interviewer: Now um, what other things that you remember as times of joy in your life, what other times would there have been?

Sophie: Well nothing stands out in my mind so much as ah, the less joyful things.

Jim was keen on fishing, and it formed a large proportion of his conversation on joy. It was with a real sense of enjoyment that he spoke of his fishing; no deep insights, but that was how Jim was – a country man, he loved the bush, but especially the river and fishing:

Interviewer: So when you look back over your life, when you look back over your life and the things you did, what things do you remember with joy? What were the best things that happened to you?

Jim: Oh well, oh gawd blimey. It's that long now I forget about it.

Interviewer: Did you do fun things with your son?

Jim: Hmm?

Interviewer: You had a son?

Jim: Yeah.

Interviewer: Did you have any other children?

Jim: Oh one, a girl. They were just as fishing mad.

Interviewer: Fishing mad, that's what you all did as a family is it?

Jim: Yeah.

Interviewer: Did your wife go fishing?

Jim: Yeah. In fact she was the one that hooked into that bloke.

Interviewer: Oh right. Yes, so she was a pretty good fisher person?

Jim: Oh she was.

Interviewer: So they were all good times were they? They were good times?

Jim: Oh yes they. Well you can see, the rivers changed on that one. Where that little bit of sand bar comes out from the other side, well I caught that big fella.

Interviewer: Hmm, very good.

Jim: Yeah, anywhere along that river I fished, anywhere and everywhere.

Simone refers to a collage prepared for her by her daughter-in-law to help her focus on the joy in her life:

> **Interviewer:** Yes that's fair enough. So as you look back over your life then, what, are they some of the things that you remember with a sense of joy? Or are there other special times that you remember with joy?
>
> **Simone:** That is 'That is Your Life'.
>
> **Interviewer:** Hmm, and that's a wonderful collage isn't it?
>
> **Simone:** Yes my daughter-in-law did that for my 90th birthday.
>
> **Interviewer:** Oh lovely, oh that's great.
>
> **Simone:** She brought it to the party. The sad part was that she didn't know I had more to fulfil the pictures of here, my first pony, my first day at work.
>
> **Interviewer:** You almost need to have another one wouldn't you, because there's a lot on that?
>
> **Simone:** Oh yes, and she put my husband and I in the centre, but there's lots of things there.

Nancy had a background in the circus. A joy in her life had been her time as a trapeze artist. She tells of her spiritual growth, learning to love herself, and then receiving the love of God into her life. She shows a sense of integrity and peace in her later life:

> **Interviewer:** As you look back over your life, what do you remember with a sense of joy?
>
> **Nancy:** Well it was a joy when I got in that circus, and got trained to be a trapeze artist and a wire walker, because I was never anything like that, I did not think I was good enough for anything.
>
> **Interviewer:** Right.
>
> **Nancy:** I never thought anything of myself.
>
> **Interviewer:** Mmm.
>
> **Nancy:** But then when I had to find out that I have to love myself.
>
> **Interviewer:** Yes.
>
> **Nancy:** First, before I could love anyone else, I looked at things and saw the love of God, and received the love of God, and it is always

there, whether I am alone, I have got the people, I can be with people or without people, I am still all that with this. I never change, I am not up and down. I am stable.

Josephine (MMSE 15) had simple memories of joy, mainly around her life as a member of a religious order:

Interviewer: And when you look back over your life and all the things that you've done, what are the things you remember with joy? What were the happy things that happened to you during your life?

Josephine: Christmas day.

Interviewer: Christmas day?

Josephine: Hmm.

Interviewer: What made that so special?

Josephine: We all got presents on Christmas day.

Interviewer: All got presents, ahh. That is special isn't it?

Josephine: Yes.

Interviewer: Any other times during your life you remember with joy?

Josephine: Going to church.

Interviewer: Going to church?

Josephine: Yes.

Interviewer: You were very committed?

Josephine: Yes.

Interviewer: Do you want to go into it a little bit?

Josephine: I'm a nun.

Interviewer: You're a nun, and what order were you in?

Josephine: Dominican.

Interviewer: Dominican nuns. You told me a little bit before about some of the things you used to do with the nuns. Can you remember what they were?

Josephine: Hmm. We had white veils, and I had to make all the veils.

Interviewer: You had to make all the veils! Hmm.

Josephine: I had to make all our veils. I could sew.

Interviewer: How old were you when you became a nun?

Josephine: I was only 16.

Interviewer: 16! Ahh. That must have been a very big decision.

Josephine: Yes, it was.

Interviewer: How did your family feel?

Josephine: Okay.

Interviewer: Okay. Were they happy?

Josephine: Yes, very happy to see me.

May remembers playing golf brought her a sense of joy. But as her conversation turns to more serious things, to her diagnosis of Alzheimer's, and then to her husband also having dementia, she may have insight into her condition and is anxious for her husband:

Interviewer: Great. What are the things that you remember with a sense of joy?

May: Oh, well, I think mainly playing golf.

Interviewer: Playing golf, yes.

May: I miss that, you know. I played tennis, and golf, but I miss, you know, not playing golf, more than anything.

Interviewer: And that was a problem with energy and actually managing to get around the course?

May: Yes, I left, no – that was just recreation, it was not a chore.

Interviewer: No, no.

May: But yes, I enjoyed that, and the company there. We have moved around a lot, my husband is in the [name] bank, and we have been moved to country towns, and I was a very, very shy person. I am not nearly as shy now, because I just had to do myself out.

Interviewer: Of course.

May: To different towns and (*pause*)...

Interviewer: Was that hard for you to do?

May: Well it was at first, but I got used to it.

Interviewer: Yes, and probably you feel good that that happened?

May: Yes I thought, think that that brought me out a lot, because I was painfully shy.

...

May: I mean he, because he was going in, and I have had Alzheimer's for five years, but has not affected me that much, but he has gone down very rapidly.

Interviewer: And has he got Alzheimer's too?

May: Yes, he's, yes. But he has only been under treatment for several months. But he was not diagnosed. His doctor would not diagnose him, so I think he is going down very quick now, because I think the medication was not in time.

Interviewer: That's a pity isn't it?

May: He's really just a shell of himself. That's a worry too.

Interviewer: That's a worry to you?

May: Yes.

Interviewer: And to him?

May: Yes, well when the family put him in here, they said I would be in later, but then they rang to say there was a bedroom next to R's [man's name] that I could I have if I came in straight away. My doctor knows that I should not be here, but it was, sort of (*pause*)...

Interviewer: It was a good time, yes. And how are you coping, living with Alzheimer's?

May: Well, I found it quite alright, it was no trouble at all, until I came in here, and I've certainly gone downhill. My memory is much worse now than when I left home, and that was only a couple of months ago.

Interviewer: Yes. Can you think of any things that might have influenced that? Was it hard coming in here, or...

May: Yes, it was really, and it is getting worse, because R [man's name] has gone downhill really quickly, he wanders at night, and into other people's rooms. He wandered in here last night, and I kept him in here for as long as I possibly could, but because it is an embarrassment. There are a lot of people in here who go around opening doors and what not, so he is not the only one, but I worry about that a lot.

Brenda was unusual among the participants in not at first being able to mention anything within either joy or sadness in her life experience:

Interviewer: That's great. Tell me, what would be the special things then, the high points, the things you remember with joy in your life? Special things.

Brenda: Don't know really. I don't think there is anything particularly special. Is there? I don't know. Never really think about it very much, do you?

Interviewer: Okay.

Brenda: I suppose the grandchildren.

Many of the participants acknowledged that their partner and/or children brought them joy, others also mentioned music, and art provided a sense of joy to some. Still others remembered travel with a sense of joy.

Summary

The spiritual dimension of wisdom has not been widely studied, even among cognitively competent older people; thus the material analysed in this study of spiritual reminiscence with people who have dementia has little basis for comparison with other older people. However, it has been exciting to examine the material from the study, looking for examples of wisdom. It is certain that numbers of the examples given from the analysed transcripts have shown some people who had significant levels of dementia, showing varying degrees of insight and the ability to grapple with difficulties of ageing and the disease of dementia. These findings are of value in combating the myths and stereotypes of dementia that would deny the possibility of these people showing any signs of wisdom, in any way.

What we were unable to demonstrate was whether those able to deal with life experiences in wise ways had developed that wisdom prior to the onset of dementia, or even through the process of dementia. Perhaps that is relatively unimportant. The findings in this area certainly raise a number of other questions for further study, for example to examine examples of a spiritual perspective of wisdom among cognitively competent older people. Another area for study is whether it might be possible to find ways of facilitating the development of wisdom in later life. Might this have implications for the well-being of older people, and perhaps even be able to raise levels of resilience and well-being in older people? It is suggested that there may be considerable overlap between wisdom and self-transcendence among these older people (see chapter 5).

8

People with Dementia in Multicultural Settings[1]

An important aspect of dementia care is the provision of culturally appropriate care. The participants in the study that forms the basis of this book were mostly Anglo-Celtic older people; however, one of the aged care facilities that was included in this project has a number of ethnic-specific residents and it was considered important to include a group of these people within the study. This chapter explores the issues of immigrants as they age and perhaps develop dementia. There is a special emphasis on one of the small spiritual reminiscence groups composed of a group of Latvian post-war migrants.

The proportion of people over the age of 65 years is continuing to increase in all OECD countries (OECD 2009). The United States, Canada, New Zealand and Australia have all been countries of high immigration, with Australia, in 2006, having the highest proportion of overseas-born people (24%), compared with New Zealand (21%), Canada (20%) and the United States (13%) (OECD 2009). In 2006, just over a quarter (27%) of Australians aged 75 years and over were born overseas (ABS 2007). Of those born overseas, 43 per cent came from other English-speaking countries, while 57 per cent were from countries where a Language Other Than English (LOTE) was the main language spoken (ABS 2007). The proportion of people with a LOTE background was higher in the 55–74 age group than in those aged over 75 years (Seebus and Peut 2010). Culture and language are both important factors to take into account when providing relevant and appropriate high-quality aged care and aged care services.

---

1 This chapter has drawn on material previously published in MacKinlay (2009).

Spirituality and ageing: Working across faiths and cultures

Context is always an important consideration in communication. MacKinlay's (2001a, 2001b) original work was done in the 1990s, within a Western society that had multicultural and multifaith components, with doctoral studies conducted with approximately half Christian people and half those of no religious affiliation, in recognition of the overall religious affiliations in Australian society. However, it is also acknowledged that the highest proportion of older people in Australia in the 1990s were of Anglo-Celtic origins. Even with the increase of immigrants from other cultures and faiths, Christianity remains the most common religion of older people in many Western societies. In the UK 2001 census, 72 per cent of people stated their religion as Christian (Office for National Statistics 2005); in the USA 47.4 per cent of census respondents described themselves as Christian church adherents[2] (US Census Bureau 2012); and in Australia 64 per cent are Christian according to recent figures (ABS 2007).

The work we have done in spirituality and reminiscence with older adults, both cognitively intact and those with dementia, has been mainly with Christians and people of no religious faith; however, the other major faith groups, those of Judaism, Islam, Buddhism and Hinduism, have growing populations of older adults, even though these numbers are still relatively small. More information on spirituality in older people of different cultures and faiths can be found in MacKinlay's, *Ageing and Spirituality Across Faiths and Cultures* (2010).

Considering these changing demographics made it important that we consider what application, if any, our work, coming out of a Christian ethos, could have for older adults of different cultures and faiths. On one level, we have been unable to conduct research in this area, even in our more recent studies; at best we have been able to access more older participants from other European countries, including Latvia and Italy. One factor in our inability to attract people of other ethnic groups may be that few of these groups of older people are residents in aged care facilities, where most of our research has been conducted. More of these people are cared for at home, by their families. This may not be so in the future as these groups of people may take on more Western styles of community life.

---

2   As the US census does not ask the question of religion, these figures cannot be accurately compared with other countries where this question is asked; it only provides numbers of people who are church adherents.

During the last two years one of us (Elizabeth) has been able to work in two Asian settings where she was able to share our work. This experience is highlighted below:

The first visit was to Singapore, where I had the opportunity to conduct a workshop with older people of different faiths and cultures and received feedback of the real relevance of my work to them. The second was about 11 days that I spent in Japan, during which time our book *Facilitating Spiritual Reminiscence for Older People with Dementia* (MacKinlay and Trevitt 2006) was launched in a Japanese translation. The book was modified with the addition of an extra chapter addressing the Christian background to the work, and with another chapter being written especially for the Japanese people to provide a context for spiritual reminiscence.

While in Japan, I had the opportunity to use spiritual reminiscence in small group work with three Japanese people who had dementia: a Catholic woman; a man who had no religious faith; and a woman with a Buddhist faith. With the assistance of a skilled translator, I was able to conduct the group, and found that the broad topics and open-ended questions that we had designed based on our research elicited similar kinds of responses from these people to those we would have expected in the original setting of the studies, yet in a different culture. I must acknowledge the high-level skill of the interpreter who had previously worked on the translation of the book. Simultaneous translation was used, and without this it would not have been possible to do this work. However, the translated process made it possible to use this material in another culture and with other faiths.

I must admit my surprise that the process we had developed worked so well, as I had been unsure whether this process of spiritual reminiscence would translate effectively to another culture. Again, I need to acknowledge the support and encouragement of the Japanese people with whom I worked. The work we did in spiritual reminiscence was filmed for a Japan Broadcasting Corporation (NHK) documentary, and in viewing this later I became aware of two important factors. First, the importance of non-verbal communication, and how my facial expressions and non-verbal cues supported the person speaking; with the simultaneous translation, there was an immediacy to the interaction, which was vital to the process. But even more so, I realised that the other two participants in the group, who also had dementia, were showing by their non-verbal engagement of body language with the person speaking of traumatic memories from earlier life that they were with her, and supporting her emotionally, as she shared. We were connecting across faiths, across cultures and in another language. This, for me, was an amazing experience.

When reflecting on the Asian experience Elizabeth found that the very questions she asked, drawn out of our original research, were questions that seemed to connect with people at a deep level even in the face of all of these differences. What we were doing was going to the core of what it is to be human. It is in effect to go beneath the cultural overlays, to ask the questions that go to the heart of being human. What does life mean? What brings joy? What brings hope? These kinds of questions go beyond national, religious and language boundaries.

So, in answer to the question 'Can spiritual reminiscence be used in other faiths and cultures?' we think the answer is 'Yes'. Of course, it is important in each context then to be sensitive to and aware of the context in which the work is being done. Respect is needed to honour and invite the participants to share; respect is fundamental to the whole process of spiritual reminiscence.

The small group of older people from Latvia

One of the spiritual reminiscence groups in this study was composed of a group of Latvians who had come to Australia during the post-war period. Although not planned this way, this homogeneous group gave a number of insights into the process and issues of ageing in a different culture. This group was one of the six-week programmes of spiritual reminiscence and certainly deserves specific consideration in this book.

Post-World War Two (WWII) immigration to Australia included many from Eastern Europe. During the period 1947–1953 more than 170,000 displaced persons arrived in Australia (Museum Victoria n.d.-a). These older ethnic groups now challenge aged care resources with cultural, language and religious issues not always understood by care providers. There were few Latvians living in Australia prior to WWII; the main immigration of close to 20,000 occurred between 1947 and 1953. These immigrants came as displaced persons under the International Resettlement Program. Few have arrived after that due to the tight controls of Soviet authorities. The average

age of this population in 2001 was 73 years (Museum Victoria n.d.-b).[3] It is said that the Latvian communities are cohesive and retain much of their culture. There are few Latvians living in the Australian Capital Territory (ACT), so they are relatively isolated from their wider cultural and community support. This is a minority ageing cultural group. The Aged Care Standards and Accreditation Agency for Australia (2008) has identified broad guidelines for the cultural and spiritual needs of aged care residents, but little study of these needs has been reported.

We wondered how this project might work for this group of older Latvians. The process of reminiscence is enjoyable for many people; however, it may also be traumatic for some. Coleman (1999) worked with Eastern European survivors of WWII, finding that where some disturbing memories remained unintegrated it was necessary to make the original experience explicit for healing to take place. Skultans (2001) was born in Latvia and returned in the 1990s with the intent of conducting a study into neurasthenia; however, this turned into an in-depth study of life story. She wrote:

> My encounter with life stories in Latvia encompassed violent and terrible events that occurred between forty and fifty years ago, the circumstances of my encounter, the setting of the narration and my informants' anxieties and hopes about the future...narrators drew upon other stories and fragments of stories to help translate a brutal chronicle into a meaningful story. (p.762)

Large numbers of Latvians experienced deportation and exile during this period; however, these exiles were determined to keep their culture and language alive following these horrific events (Skultans 2001). The power of these early experiences in a hostile environment was clearly expressed by participants in this group of older Latvians, when they were invited to be part of this study. Perhaps not surprisingly, the participants were at first suspicious of the motives of the researchers. These suspicions were in contrast to the readiness of other participants to take part in the study. This group of older people were especially concerned about the possibility of their names being used and the use of the tape-recorder. Extra care was taken to explain and reassure participants about the reasons for the study and their contribution. The participants were deemed to have a good understanding of English; therefore translation services were not required. Previously these

---

3   Demographics from the State of Victoria were chosen as this was the largest Latvian settlement in Australia, and it is likely that most of the study group reported in this chapter came from the Victorian settlement, even though the members of the study group were resident in the ACT.

residents had kept largely to themselves in the care facility, rarely engaging in the activities provided for residents. A second and practical difficulty in the study was that the transcribers often found it difficult to understand the participants' accents on the audio-tapes.

One participant asked why we were interested in Latvia. It was explained that it was not primarily Latvia that we were interested in, but their lives. However, as the groups progressed through the weekly sessions, it became apparent that being Latvian was indeed an important component of their identity, and therefore provided an important insight into how they were ageing and the effects of culture and their early life experiences on their well-being now.

To help overcome the frailty and communication difficulties experienced by this group, it was limited to three participants. Their ages ranged from 87 to 94 years, with Mini Mental State Examination (MMSE) scores of 18–20. Two of the three participants had lived together before entering the aged care facility. All three shared a common first language, culture and religious denomination (Lutheran). They had not been involved in any group that supported reminiscence of these early life events whilst at the aged care facility. Despite this, they were eager to share their memories, even in the face of dementia and English as a second language.

Meaning in life

Sophia said her singing had given her greatest meaning (she was an opera singer); however, lack of money for her training meant that she was only ever in the chorus. Sophia showed the group facilitator a patchwork quilt on her knees that she had made (it was beautiful), and the facilitator attended to it, touching it as Sophia spoke. Sophia told the group that her mother died when she was three. Her older sister looked after her and taught her to read from the newspaper.

Sophia likes poetry: 'I do, I do a lot.' She said that she had it here (the poetry she has written), about 75 pages of it, and suddenly it disappeared. She was visibly upset by this. She said that she cried and cried. She said that she asked her daughter if she took it and she said no. It was all the time in her drawer, but now it is gone. It was in Latvian, so she can't understand why someone else would have taken it. She has read it to a woman in the kitchen, and she said it was beautiful. (It seems she translated it.)

Phillip spoke about his work here, but not back in Latvia. He was a soldier, in the German army. He said: 'My father died when I was seven years old.' Then, he told of being caught in the war. Here, in a new country after the war, he said nobody liked him – not the Germans, not the Australians. He talked about being in a concentration camp. At another point he remembered the summer festivals in Latvia where they sang and danced all night. He smiled for some time at the memory, and that he had been involved in something adventurous. He did not normally show much emotion.

Emily wanted to see a copy of the questions, which were on the table in the middle of the group. She read them and laughed out loud, saying, 'How can you answer these? It is impossible.' But she began to answer anyway, on the question of 'What keeps you going?' She talked about 'mental and metaphysical' concerns as the hardest to deal with, and about keeping herself occupied. She spoke of how happy she has been in her life, good and well looked-after, and very happy to be here in Australia. She laughed again at the impossibility of answering the questions. She said that she was in two wars. She escaped from WWII and came to Australia. She talked of the war – she was in Latvia caught between the Russian army on one side and the German army on the other. She reported that she was not injured during her escape. She spoke again of being grateful to Australia; then she broke down and cried.

Connectedness and relationships

In the groups of participants in the larger study, all with dementia, an important finding was their need for connectedness with others. This was the case for this group as well, even though at times some found this need hard to express. Sophia remarked:

> I have friends and still, here in Australia and, but they are still alive, but lost, lost. A couple of months, and she came here for my birthday, on Wednesday, I can't remember now. Sometimes my tragedy with my health, or a lot of things going around, I could not understand.

She seemed to be expressing her aloneness in the words 'still alive, but lost, lost'. A significant time for visiting was her birthday, which she has difficulty placing in a context of time. Then Sophia seemed to show insight into her confusion, in the last sentence of the quote above. Sophia went on to speak of dreams, and her husband. 'Yes, terrible dreams, sometimes very good dreams, when my husband came over and speak with me, and thank me, and...'

GRIEF

Grief formed an important sub-theme of connectedness and relationship during the group sessions. Emily talked about her husband's death in their second year in Australia. Her husband was a builder, and had not had his tetanus injection, and died following an accident. She cried as she told this. She was in a new country, she could not speak English, and their daughter was only about five years old. She became quite upset as she remembered these events, from so long ago.

Sophia said that she has lost too much. The observer notes from the session revealed that she sat hunched over with her head down as she spoke these words. But Sophia also talked of her health problems and hoped that she got better 'from my leg' (she is now wheelchair-bound). She had many sad memories – when her husband died. She struggled for words (against her dementia, and in English as a foreign language) to speak of her love of craft and embroidery, and the sadness at the loss of these. As she spoke she got more and more upset, fiddling with her handbag on her lap, sitting hunched forward, and at this point began to cry. She continued to speak, crying as she talked. She talked of dressmaking, and although tears were still running down her face, she looked brighter and seemed to have more energy.

LONELINESS
Another sub-theme of connectedness and relationship was loneliness. Sophia was sometimes lonely. She spoke of her terrible dreams that she had at night. She mostly doesn't like being alone. Her mind is too busy, goes 'up and around'.

In response to the question about being alone, Phillip said, 'Oh, yes.' And he explained, it was mostly when he woke up. But he didn't mind being alone at times.

LANGUAGE DIFFICULTIES AND SENSE OF ISOLATION
Sophia said:

> I sit down and my lady who comes with me, and she said, 'Why didn't you speak?', but my mind keeps going up around and around and I really don't nothing what to do with her, because she has different, has different, she is different, she does not speak in our language.

Sophia was able to express her concern that the volunteer who came to visit her didn't speak her language. Sophia was doubly disadvantaged, with English as her second language and dementia that made it difficult for her to express herself in English. This resulted in Sophia becoming even more isolated within the aged care facility.

The group facilitator asked Phillip: 'And nobody else from your church or anyone comes to see you?' Phillip replied: 'No, except the congregation.' It is hard to know whether his response is lack of understanding of the question, perhaps related to his dementia, or lack of understanding of the spoken English.

Spiritual and religious practices

The three people in this group with dementia shared deeply about their image of God and God's place in their lives. It is interesting to contrast the answer that Phillip gave in the quotation in the last paragraph above and his discussion about his understanding of God that follows. In the following quotations he is able to express complex concepts meaningfully. Phillip explained his continuing relationship with God, saying: 'God is everything involved with daily life.'

On the question of what he thought God was like, Phillip said:

> I think that question really, can, that is such question that you can think and say that, but really answer if you can the question. It is very, very deep. That not mine, we know it is knowledge, but is not freely in use, it is knowledge to remind you about something, but the feeling is God is something we know, absolute something.

Phillip expanded on his understanding of God: 'I believe in something, but not that God is a man or something walking around the street, I can't explain what it is, but it is something, being over our mind and over our lives.'

Emily explained her relationship with God through saying, 'I find it by reading the Bible.'

Sophia said:

> But I think the highest, not the church, or the priest, you can listen, but that is still yours. That is very deep question, it really can't be answered. One thing, that is another, but there is a time for everything, there is one who do you express it, but that is how I feel that way, that's what I wanted to say. God is the same because we pray with our soul, that is the same and that's what is with God.

Again, Sophia, as well as Phillip, showed a depth of understanding and appreciation of the nature of God and their relationship with God. This understanding expressed is one of a maturity of faith that is more likely in old age (Fowler 1981).

Emily said:

> And sometimes I feel yes, I did much when I said other parts they don't know, but I did, I did believe it, I did but, and I feel my heart is much better and then I come close my eyes and I can say thank you, thank you to God, thank you to Jesus for helping me, because that is what… That is how I think from my life, I have been through all of this, I have been walking long, for many hundreds and thousands nights, and I hear the children cry, and I feel alright, and he saves us, he saves us, not the sky is falling or anything.

Emily reflected on times gone by, when she was young, and her faith that sustained her then in times of trouble and distress, and she noted that same faith still supported her.

In the context of conversation about what it was like to live in wartime, the topic turned to the difficulty of religious practices. Phillip reflected on experiences of war, again with a theme of trauma, but faith sustaining them – knowing that God was near:

> If I think in my head, in my heart, then you told, you live and come, going on, and it's just hells, you know, this pleading, and that is not right, when you just go and say for now, but I love my God and thanks God for that. If I had, in the war, then the night when the bombs was coming down and we feel, we feel an old man sitting behind, and my children was lying down, and she was sleeping, and I take my arms and I said 'My God, don't do that. Think what about the children', and I heard the bombs, it was one home, a little bit worse, so that means that I was believing, I was believing, when God was with us, he is always there, God is with us. Thank you.

Vulnerability and transcendence

About growing older, Emily said: 'You have to accept it, you are always growing old, not, oh you can choose it, that's the only way.'

Sophia said: 'I do everyday work that I can do, but I can't, yesterday I was trying to walk, but… I will walk, I walk good maybe from one to two doors, but that is not real walking, that is terrible.'

Phillip expressed his attitude to life in the following way:

I am over 90 years, and in these 90 years…that is things you can't explain, no one can explain. Different, but I thank the Lord I am still alive, thank the Lord, I am happy I am still alive, there is a moment when you think that you would be better if you not alive, and that I can't explain.

These participants were showing signs of resiliency and transcendence in their later lives. They seemed to cope well with adversity. It is apparent that there is some association with their long history of war and dislocation in earlier life, but its extent is unknown.

Sometimes the group members really supported each other, as they understood the meanings of these remembered stories and the traumas of the past far better than any outsider could have done. This inner cultural wisdom and understanding would have set these people apart from others in the facility, and apart from staff who had no common history with them. This common cultural experience of the group members could not have been bridged simply by translation of language; it went far deeper than that. Perhaps this was a real strength of the group sessions for these participants. Would group sessions over a longer term work better in supporting these people? Overall in the larger study, the longer groups showed stronger outcomes for group interaction and cohesiveness. It is hard to say whether this particular group would have benefited from being in a long-term group. The group interactions of spiritual reminiscence over the six weeks showed the potential for supporting older people from Eastern European countries in processing traumatic memories. Simply sharing these memories in a supported environment seemed beneficial.

Further staff education will be important for increasing awareness of the issues and form a means for improving support for older people of different ethnic backgrounds. These issues will become more prominent as groups of displaced persons from WWII grow still older and need residential care. Issues of language, faith and culture, interlaced with memories of trauma, will become important aspects of care for these elderly people.

The communication style of the facilitator is important in every setting, and in each setting it is important that the facilitator is able to connect with the particular group that he or she guides. The facilitator in this instance brought her own mix of skills to the project. Moving on from topics before participants were able to process what was being said was particularly a problem for this culturally and linguistically diverse group of people. Failing to pick up on cues from participants was another problem. One suggestion from a participant would have assisted the facilitator: 'Oh, I not prepared for this question. Write a couple of questions on paper, and when are you here, write them, please, but sometimes I do not know. There are too many things what I think is important.' This was a particular issue in understanding written versus spoken language, and in particular for people with dementia.

Overall, we felt that the six-week group session was very short for these older people with dementia, struggling with a different language and culture. Would it have been valuable to continue the group for longer? The research plan was to use six-week groups for those with particular problems, and the language problems of this group, coupled with their dementia, made this a somewhat challenging group. We note the suspicions that some of the group expressed before the groups began, about the reasons for the research and protection of their privacy. However, during the sessions, they shared generously and demonstrated deep understandings of their lives, and the ways they coped with growing losses and the disabilities of ageing. Issues of war traumas and memories, and hard experiences when they were young, kept coming back into the conversations. The participants also showed wisdom and deep understandings of their faith.

Summary

Australia is a multicultural country, and this means that as our migrant population ages they will face significant challenges. In aged care facilities there are very few carers who speak a language other than English, and so those for whom English is a second language may struggle to be understood as their dementia deepens. Although predominantly a Christian country, there are significant numbers of people of other faiths living in Australia. We have found from our group of Latvian participants and from Elizabeth's experience in Asia that spiritual reminiscence can cross the cultural divide and capture issues of ageing and dementia.

9

Hope and Despair among Those with Dementia

The battle for recognising the *person* with dementia has been going on now for at least the last couple of decades. But now, there seems to be new light dawning on a much wider sphere of dementia care and well-being. In our spiritual reminiscence groups, participants clearly articulated their hopes for the future. Participants spoke of sad times, but they were generally able to overcome these difficulties in their lives.

A change of practice and public policy: New hope for people with dementia

It is encouraging to see that public policy is shifting to take a positive approach to care with people who have dementia (Wolverson, Clarke and Moniz-Cook 2010). The language has changed to include an emphasis on rehabilitation of people with dementia, not simply dealing with 'dementia-sufferer behaviours'. This in itself is a great sign of hope for people who have dementia and their loved ones, and indeed for all who provide care. Just a few years ago, there was no sign of any possibility of a positive approach to dementia. Tom Kitwood was among the first to recognise the 'malignant psychology of dementia' (1997), a term he used to describe the way that dementia was portrayed through the dominant paradigm of medicine, that disempowered and thus robbed the person of their very personhood.

However, the major emphasis in care and treatment remained firmly based in this mould of the biomedical model until quite recently. Some other important work that has helped to break down the barriers to people with dementia being accepted as still being people has come from courageous individuals who were themselves diagnosed with dementia (e.g. Boden 1998); people who were able to articulate clearly what it was like to have this diagnosis and live with the stereotypes that often regarded them as 'non-persons'. But things are changing; there is new hope, as more people – including: professional healthcare providers across a wide variety of disciplines; people with dementia; and practical theologians – address a common theme of finding the best means of affirming and enabling people who have dementia to live the best and most fruitful lives possible.

Evidence of this new hope is also apparent in the wider professional literature, with a recent article in *The Lancet* on the death of the great researcher and writer Robert Butler, titled 'The art of medicine: Overcoming the social death of dementia through language' (George 2010). This article addresses the changes that produced a picture of cognitive decline in later life as a disease to be cured, just as polio had been a disease to be beaten some decades before. It outlines the four decades of 'war on Alzheimer's' that followed. It is acknowledged that this approach did result in increased funding in search of a cure not for dementia but for 'Alzheimer's', as the new name came to the forefront of popular usage. What this approach to any type of dementia failed to do was to remove the fear of the disease; in fact, it would be fair to say that fear of the disease was increased over this time. It is hard to find hope in the midst of beliefs of loss of self as dementia progresses and predictions of a tsunami of future cases of dementia.

In a hopeful contrast, within this article, the author notes that the person's identity is never completely lost until death, and that a more empathetic attitude is needed 'for changes in personhood rather than stoking fear and sadness, and [to] guide attention towards the remaining humanity in those with dementia and the means through which they can be meaningfully included in the activities of our daily lives' (George 2010, p.587). These changing attitudes bring a real sense of hope into this field at an important time.

What is hope?

Hope is both personal and communal. A whole community can be infused with hope, inspired to give and be of its best. Individuals can be hopeful or hopeless. It seems that there can be movement between the communal expectations of hope and the individual's expectations of hope. Some individuals can hold hope, even in the face of societal despair. It is worth mentioning that the other side of hope is despair and hopelessness.

In a secular sense, hope is seen in the person who holds on to life and refuses to give up, for example an elderly person who sees that life is worth living; that there is still meaning in life. In a humanistic sense, hope comes from within the person and is associated with the person's belief in their own abilities. Hope in the Christian context is, in Paul's words from Colossians 1:27, the mystery of the riches of the glory of God, 'which is Christ in you, the hope of glory'. Hope is portrayed among people of faith of the Abrahamic religions through their scriptures, ritual and doctrines and the beliefs by which they live their lives. For most, there is a belief in some kind of after-life, which gives a sense of hope of things to come, not only focusing on the things of this life. Buddhists and Hindus also see hope in their religious scriptures and beliefs that assert the continuity of life; and thus hope can be seen in the continuing cycle of life, death and renewed life.

Yet hope as it stands in the present and its 'statements of promise, however, must stand in contradiction to the reality which can at present be experienced' (Moltmann 1967, p.18). Indeed, it was this kind of hope that Frankl (1984) saw among those who survived the concentration camp experiences of WWII; he observed the survival of people who experienced horrific torture, people who hoped for something that they could not hold at that time, except in their hearts and wills – for example the hope to be reunited with a loved one after the war was over. On the other hand, Frankl also witnessed the death of those experiencing the same tortures, but who had no sense of hope. It is important, of course, to distinguish between the reality of hope on the one hand and, on the other, the wishful thinking or denial involved in short-term defence mechanisms (Wolverson *et al.* 2010). Hope is based on reality as perceived by the person, even though there might not be physical evidence to support the hope. There is a sense in which hope seeks what has not yet been fully grasped by the person. Moltmann expresses this by saying, 'They seek…to lead existing reality towards the promised and hoped-for transformation.' Hope is expressed in Romans 8: 24–25, where Paul writes that we are saved by hope, but hope that is seen is not hope; rather it is a present waiting and trusting of things to come. As Moltmann writes, 'Christian hope is resurrection hope' (Moltmann 1967, p.18).

Hopelessness

In contrast to hope, hopelessness is closely associated with suicide, and this is no less so in later life. In fact, rates of completed suicide are higher among older men, and Gulbinat (cited in De Leo *et al.* 2001) noted that when the 15–24 age group is compared with the 75+ age group, suicide is up to seven times more likely among the 75+ group. Often among older people, death through suicide is regarded quite differently from the tragedy of youth suicide. It is often said of the older person, 'Well he had lived a good long life.' Sometimes late-life suicide is described as rational suicide, in that suicide in late life is seen as a reasonable choice in the face of the loss of meaning in older people. Hope is closely tied to finding meaning in one's existence, and it is often assumed that there is no meaning in the life of older people, as the ability to retain control over one's life is diminished, and skills and capacities are lost. Yet, as has been recorded in other chapters in this book, especially in the chapter on resilience and transcendence, meaning can be found, even in the face of disability and loss. If meaning can be found, hope can exist.

Hope and people with dementia

We began these studies because of the need to see how people with dementia could find meaning in this experience of dementia. Of course, meaning is closely associated with hope; without meaning, there is no hope. It is well known that depression is often associated with dementia. Depression can obviously negatively affect the possibility of hope, and we searched the literature to find examples that might help explain the situation for people with dementia and hope. In a three-year study 114 patients with mild cognitive dysfunction were divided into two groups based on 'whether or not they also showed depressive symptoms' (Kasahara et al. 2006). The study found that 'dementia developed in 33% of the patients with no depressive symptoms, but in 85% of the patients with depressive symptoms' (p.129). This corroborates the finding of a five-year follow-up study of life events and survival in dementia by Butler et al. (2004): 'the only psychiatric or social factor associated with poor survival in dementia was depression' (p.702). If we were able to find ways of assisting people with dementia to find meaning, this may also assist with lowering depression, and thus indirectly this would make a difference in their outlook of hope, or hopelessness.

Herth (1990) defined hope as 'an inner power directed toward enrichment of "being"', and developed a multidimensional hope scale to assess hopefulness in nursing settings. Herth (1992) has set out to capture the multidimensional nature of hope, noting that hope is composed of an interpersonal element, a time-oriented sense, a future focus and a goal-achievement expectation. To these previously identified dimensions of hope, Herth has added the following:

- a more global, non-time-oriented sense of hope
- hope despite diminished or absent interpersonal relationships
- hope as a sense of 'being' available and engaging in relationships, as opposed to 'doing' for oneself and others
- potential of hope for controlling behavioural or emotional responses, as opposed to the control of events or experiences.

Herth developed her original Herth Hope Scale into the Herth Hope Index (HHI) (Herth 1992, 2005), a 12-item Likert scale for use with frail and elderly clients, especially in palliative care, with the particular aim of identifying issues of hope in clinical settings. The elements of the index pick up on issues of a spiritual dimension and go some way towards identifying the complexity of this important construct. While our study of spiritual reminiscence taps into meaning for the participants in the small group sessions, and is a longitudinal project, not a clinical assessment, it is useful to compare the content of the HHI with the issues that were raised by the participants in our work. Buckley and Herth (2004) reported from an earlier study that 'terminally ill patients defined hope as "an inner power that facilitates the transcendence of the present situation and movement toward new awareness and enrichment of being"' (p.36). This is very much a spiritual perspective on hope, as discussed in this chapter. MacKinlay's (2001a) model of the spiritual tasks and process of ageing sees hope associated with relationship, the ability for transcendence, and finding meaning, again assuming multifaceted aspects to the concept of hope.

Wolverson *et al.* (2010) studied hope among people with early dementia. Using the concept of rehabilitation, they examined how this can be used to maximise the well-being of people with dementia. An important finding from their study was that comparison between the literature on hope with people without dementia, and their study of people with dementia, did not show any real differences between the groups. More and more we are gaining evidence that people who have dementia still have the same hopes and needs as other people; this is important news in societies where there are high levels of people fearful of those who have dementia. In comparing their study with that of two other studies of older people, Wolverson *et al.* noted that, specifically in those without dementia, there was a

> relative absence of future-orientated goals relating to 'the self' and the apparent absence of hoped 'for' achievements, goals, or outcomes (Farran, Salloway and Clark, 1990; Herth, 1993). In explaining the first of these, we suggest that older people may have their own unique interpretation of the future. (p.456)

They note that their data fitted with the presence of 'world-related goals' found by others in older people, and reflects the importance of meaning and integrity in later life. They note, too, the desire to pass on a 'legacy of hope' to the next generation. Thus they saw that the absence of goal attainment in their older participants was evidence of a generalised rather than particularised type of hope. Further, Wolverson *et al.* (2010) noted differences between optimism and hope among the limited number of studies of older people and hope, and found that, among the study participants who had early-stage dementia, the 'construct of optimism may be less relevant' than the construct of hope (p.456), given the relative absence of goal-attainment outcomes hoped for. They also suggest that the more generalised hope of these people with dementia may assist in preserving meaning. In conclusion, noting the need for further study, and for hope-affirming support measures, Wolverson *et al.* (2010) found:

> In older people with and without dementia, increased infirmity, impairments and/or losses, and an assumed need for greater reliance on others are described as potential barriers to hope. However, dementia-specific barriers to hope were also evident, in the attitudes of others and experiences of loss of role, loss of respect, and no longer being listened to. (p.457)

Thus, in their study, it was not dementia that specifically influenced hope, but hope was also associated with effects of ageing and was similar to hope expressed by other older people, without dementia. In our study, we had a range of levels of dementia among the participants; while they only had people with early dementia, our participants were all in need of residential care due to their dementia. So does hope still continue to be of a similar form for these people? We show examples from our study in the remainder of this chapter.

Participants sometimes raised loss of memory as a concern, and Jessica (MMSE 9) connected memory with retaining hope in her life.

Interviewer: You don't know, okay. And what gives you hope in life now?

Jessica: Hope?

Interviewer: Yep.

Jessica: Memory.

Interviewer: Memory?

Jessica: Yes.

Interviewer: Tell me about that.

Jessica: Remembering things.

Interviewer: That gives you hope, remembering things?

Jessica: Yes.

Interviewer: So you try and remember things?

Jessica: Keep playing them to retain them.

Interviewer: Keep playing the memories back. So that is really participating in life, isn't it?

Jessica: Yes.

Examples of hope from the study

In this study, there were many examples of hope among the comments and discussions of these people with dementia. It may be asked, to what degree are these people, often with low cognitive abilities (MMSE levels varying from 4 to several at 30, with mean MMSE of 18, but all diagnosed with dementia), able to engage with hope? It is apparent through the evidence of the topics of discussion that these people did know what hope was about. Often they engaged with questions of hope on the basis of hoping for good things for their children and grandchildren, just as other older people do. But there was also much more; we will use their words to share through the transcripts of sessions and interviews where they find hope in the experience of dementia.

Prayer

Anticipation of prayers answered was one way in which hope was expressed in small group sessions. This provided an assurance for these people with dementia; for example, see Joyce's statement below.

Joyce: Just doing what I can for my family, and uh, more or less is the main thing, that gives me hope, and my prayers, yes. I always, well I have a belief and I think my prayers are answered, so that's why I pray my prayers.

In an in-depth interview, Bob explained that he found hope through his prayers:

Interviewer: What is it that gives you hope now?

Bob: What is it that I hope now?

Interviewer: Yes. What is it, where do you find hope now?

Bob: Um, well I find hope in my prayers, ah that I can live a reasonably long life. Err, end of story.

Interviewer: Okay.

In another in-depth interview, Mavis saw hope as part of her everyday journey with the Lord, completed in prayer in the evening of each day:

> **Mavis:** I think the hope is, when I say my night prayers, I just get into bed, and say, you know, a bit of a resume, of my day, and uh, as if the Lord doesn't know it, and then I say, right I am going to sleep now.

Sense of acceptance

A sense of acceptance of life and all that it brings was clearly evident in the comments of some participants. Being ready to die was one such example and was seen in some group members. This acceptance of forthcoming death did not seem to be one of resignation, but of being ready to face this final part of life.

> **Facilitator:** What gives you hope now?
>
> **Hetty:** Well, I am ready to go. I have lived all my life. And I am not worried about going.

In another group session the following conversation took place:

> **Facilitator:** Wonderful, that's wonderful. Okay. A number of these things we have actually talked about it, various things already, right, well, what is it that gives you hope in life now?
>
> **Daphne:** Oh, only that.
>
> **Facilitator:** Only that?
>
> **Daphne:** Yes. Well, I mean I have achieved, I feel I have achieved all I can achieve in this world, that is how I feel. I have worked hard at many professions and, or just ordinary blue-collar work if you like, put it that way. I have worked in factories, I have been successful in that, and had control of a room full of people working making shoes, and over here I was in the public service, I came back alright after all that ordeal, got back and did more and more examinations, as you do, to go up the ladder as it were, and that is how I did, and I got promotions to, a promotion to Sydney, after eight years being in Hobart, and I was only there six years, and somebody from Canberra learnt I was studying, what is the name of the course, ah, not bookkeeping, more than that, the whole…

Elvie shows through her responses that she may not have wanted to be living in an aged care facility, but now that she is, she had accepted this and is making the most of it. At the same time, she admits to being content being alone: 'I'm a real loner.' Elvie attributed her acceptance to 'I've got that sort of nature', showing insight into her ways of coping and personality.

Interviewer: What gives you hope in life now?

Elvie: Hope? I don't seem to need hope do I? What's hope for, to hope you're going to do something? I'm quite content what I'm, where I am, but I have to be really, but I'm lucky I've got that sort of nature. You know I didn't want to come here, but I accept it and make myself happy. I don't mix a lot, I'm a real loner, but er yes. I say most. That's my favourite spot out there that I'm sort of cleaning and planting at the moment.

In her in-depth interview, Loretta, in contrast, seems not to have given the subject of hope a great deal of thought. Yet it seemed that she accepted her life for what it was.

Loretta: I don't bother with hope, I don't think. Sometimes I hope for the outcome of something that is being done, but there is nothing in particular, I don't wish for anything that I have not got.

Acceptance may simply be related to having a sense of safety and security, as in this example below. This was an important issue related to fear among independent-living older people (MacKinlay 2001a), which was much diminished among frail older, cognitively intact people in another study (MacKinlay 2006). Numbers of older people in the study of frail older people remarked that they were no longer fearful, as they felt that someone would come if they had a need; they felt secure. In the excerpt below, Stella (MMSE 8) says she feels at home and safe:

Interviewer: And what things give you hope now?

Stella: Well the thing is, first and foremost I have been, I feel safe here.

Interviewer: So feeling safe is really important.

Stella: Mmm, I feel safe, it does not matter, I feel safe. And that whatever's to be, or what have you, I am here and I am safe. That's how I feel, you know, I don't want to do this, that or anything else, if anything can help with it I like to do that, but thing is I feel I am home and safe.

Brenda shows a real sense of serenity in her reply:

Interviewer: Good. Now, what about hope in your life? What do you hope for now?

Brenda: Nothing really. Nothing extra. Everything I need.

Interviewer: Everything you need you have. Good.

Brenda: Lucky aren't I?

Interviewer: You are, yes.

Brenda: Very lucky.

Faith

Some participants spoke of the support that their faith brought them. First, examples from in-depth interviews:

Daphne: The future for me is to go and, uh, at one time, when He is ready, uh, put me into, um, a place that He has prepared for me.

Interviewer: What gives you hope now?

Graham: My hope for the Lord is do the best I can with what I have got.

Interviewer: Yep.

Graham: And I can't do any more than that, and my goal was because, because of their problems, they have got to work, some of them have got to work with me, not that I am a teacher or anything, but I have been doing a bit of relieving sometimes, and because I, because I did that, it gave me, it pushed me into other little realms.

Interviewer: Mmm.

Graham: And then, if it's Saturday or Sunday night I will sit down and read that chapter, and I find that a great help, and wonder how my speech is. Are you? (*both laugh*)

Interviewer: Okay, now is there any way that we can help you find meaning in life now?

Graham: Oh, yes I can, I can find meaning in life, I have the capacity now.

Interviewer: Yes.

Graham: To understand what it is about. I did not know, I could put, I could put 20 verses in a, and it couldn't mean as much to me as what it would, as what it did, knowing the both of us. And we worked together.

In the following examples are a number of instances from the small groups reflecting on hope and their faith:

Eve: I suppose I want to be the person that I would choose to be.

Facilitator: Yes.

Eve: Uh, I mean we can't all do the things the right way I know, but I would like to be, uh, I don't think I would want to be a great biblical, you know, reader or whatever, but I would like to, do my bit for God, you know, and, or for anyone, if there was a need for, you know, support for someone or something like that.

Graham: My hope for the Lord is, do the best I can with what I have got.

Facilitator: What gives you hope, now?

Candy: Christianity I think, that is a hope. My hope, other people have different ideas.

Facilitator: So what is it that gives you hope in life now?

Nancy: I am just hoping to meet as many people as I can, uh to, to get this message through, because I know that God means me to do it. I know what He wants. And death, I just wait, because He said those who wait upon the Lord will rise up like an eagle.

Still wanting to engage with life

It was evident that a number of these participants still wanted to engage with life as fully as they could. Some had realistic hopes, but others held on to unrealistic hopes and dreams, yet felt comfortable with these. Participants often hoped for good health; one wanted to go on a cruise; and yet another had sight problems but felt happy and contented.

Interviewer: And what gives you hope now?

Don: As I said, to complete some of the things that I set out to do, which needs to be done, not for my sake so much as for the people directly concerned.

Facilitator: Mmm.

Don: And look forward to being, you know, satisfactory completed. And I hope I can maintain a decent health so I am not a burden to anyone else.

Interviewer: As you get closer to the end of your life now, what do you look forward to?

Candy: Uh, I would not mind going on a cruise to tell you the truth, to NZ, just a short cruise or something like that, but I don't know if it is possible, but I would like to.

Interviewer: So you would like to do a bit more travel would you?

Candy: Yes, just a cruise, I enjoy cruises. It's, yes, that's about all I look forward to. And as much time with the family I can get, and talking to people.

Interviewer: So what is it, um, that gives you hope in life now?

Bronwyn: I hope to be able to continue on in life for a little while, helping anyone that I can.

Interviewer: Yes.

Bronwyn: I know that I have very poor eyesight now, that's because I'm old. But otherwise I feel very happy and contented.

Fear of future suffering

Fear of future suffering was an important topic for cognitively competent independent-living older people. It is interesting that, when we looked for this theme in these participants, it did not feature in the topics that they raised. Was this because they were not aware of the future? Was it because they had no fears? There were actually few fears mentioned.

Family

Concerns for children and grandchildren and the future were a common topic for these people. This topic is dealt with in more detail in chapter 13. First, from the in-depth interviews:

Lotty: The future generations. I have, in some people more than others. I have one nephew starting medicine this year; I think he'll be a wonderful doctor. And my hope is, my hope is with him. Hope not to be a nuisance to the family. Hope to see family more often.

Una: I'm just hoping that I eventually can manage to be away from here on my own somewhere to be near my family.

Interviewer: Mmm hmm. What gives you hope now?

Louise: Hope?

Interviewer: Hope.

Louise: Well I would not be doing anything really, because I know my three sons are all here, you know, and I like this here, yes.

Interviewer: So your life really is very much focused on those three sons now, isn't it?

Louise: Something?

Interviewer: Your life is very much centred on your three boys?

Louise: Yes, it is. Well you can see up there where they (*pause*)...

Interviewer: Yes, heaps of photos of them. They look lovely.

Louise: They are very young there, really.

Interviewer: Yes, yes. You have got lots of lovely photos around here.

Louise: Yes, it's very good really.

Interviewer: And what gives you hope in life now?

Mary: Err, that I won't be a nuisance to the family.

Interviewer: Okay, what gives you hope in life now?

Anita: Sometimes I lose it a bit.

Interviewer: Do you?

Anita: I just think of what's going to happen when I'm gone, but I can't alter that can I?

Interviewer: No.

Anita: Otherwise I don't really worry about things and I don't worry them. I don't want to go and live with them because they've got their wife and children and I don't think it's fair to the wives and so they come on Sunday and they take me out for dinner and that sort of thing.

Interviewer: That's good.

Anita: Otherwise I'm sorry that I can't (*unfinished*)

Eunice took time to begin to speak of family, but what she had to say then was both important and difficult (see below). Sometimes simply being able to share these things with another person who listens with respect and gives time to the speaker is all that is needed for supporting the speaker.

Eunice: But at 90, why wouldn't I? What can I look forward to at 90?

Interviewer: Well. That's what I'm asking you. Um, what gives you hope in life now?

Eunice: What gives me hope in life now? What gives me hope? For my daughter [name]. She's got a dreadful back, and she's going to end up an absolute cripple, and err God's not there, that's all. That shocks you I bet.

Interviewer: No. It doesn't shock me, I've heard it times before. Um, is there anything else about the spiritual journey of life that you want to tell me?

Eunice: No.

Una still longs to be near her family, and she is struggling with adjustment to living in this setting. We found on a number of occasions that these people might have said they had only just arrived at this facility, but staff confirmed they had been there for some months, or longer. Cognitive decline can lead to differences in perception of time.

Interviewer: And what gives you hope now?

Una: I'm just hoping that I eventually can manage to be away from here on my own somewhere to be near my family. At my age, although they're very kind to me here, but they've been very good to me, I've only been here a couple of weeks, I don't know how long it is, but it's not very long that I've been here. My family came to see me, but I'd like to be well enough to get back to family.

The following participant, Edith, had an MMSE of just 5. She spoke about her mother, and while the memory of her mother was clear, she had no perception of time. Her mother had certainly not been cooking for many years, and would have been dead for a long time. However, the memory of that relationship was still of significance to Edith and could still be affirmed appropriately by those who cared for her.

Interviewer: What gives you hope now?

Edith: Well, because my mother is still alive, which is wonderful. She is a wonderful lady and she has a wonderful thing for cooking.

Interviewer: Mmm hmm.

Edith: She does wonderful cooking. And uh, I have never stuck to, or said anything but not to do it, or anything like that, and she has always done it, down the pages, as you can see now. And she, she is always, loved her piano. I think it was because it was my mother.

No sense of hope, resignation

Some participants could not see hope in their lives. This is not necessarily related to the dementia, but may also be associated with personality and other factors related to growing older. The first participant below, in an in-depth interview, sees no hope in life yet seems to accept in a determined way to continue to live, without any perceived source of hope. There is also a sense of self-sacrifice in this account where Margaret kept the fact of not wanting to be admitted to this place a secret from her children, seeing that 'for the best'. She also recognised her increasing frailty, shown by the fall and subsequent fracture. This is a hard decision, made by many older people. Loraine, in her interview, voiced her sense of no longer finding any meaning in life. Spiritual reminiscence may assist some of these people to find meaning, even in their current situation. It may mean pastorally working with the person, one-on-one, if the person is willing. Sharing their story, in depth, may prove helpful.

Margaret: Well there's no hope.

Interviewer: There's no hope?

Margaret: I've just got to go on. Hmm, that's what I think anyhow. The family have put me here, I didn't want to come, but I didn't tell them that. This is the best I think. Because I fall over. I fell and broke my wrist and that started it all off.

Interviewer: Yes and you really feel that you can't manage by yourself any more.

Margaret: No.

Interviewer: Yeah it's a hard decision isn't it?

Margaret: Hmm. Yes it is, it is a hard decision, but once you've made it you've got to go through with it I think.

Interviewer: Um, well what gives you hope for the future?

Loraine: I have none. I have no hope for anything now.

Interviewer: No hope for the future?

Loraine: Gone. It isn't there. I have none.

May, in the excerpt below, clearly expressed her belief that at 80 years of age she had lived long enough, and there was no hope left; life was over. She seemed to be associating hope with activity, in what she used to be able to do, and had obviously not transcended into a 'being' mode in later life. It seems that failure to move towards transcendence forms a real block to further letting go and the possibility of spiritual growth in the face of adversity. In the excerpt below, it is interesting that when the interviewer began to ask and explore what other things might be possible, May did not want to go further, nor did she seem open to other possibilities. A clue to her enjoyment of playing bridge might be the mention she made of her friends, who she obviously misses.

Interviewer: That's good. What brings you hope in life now?

May: I haven't any really, I just think it's over. I, you know, had 80 years and that's enough, really, so I don't look forward to anything. Lived a really active life, I played bridge. I miss that. I played right up until I came up here.

Interviewer: Oh, I wonder if there is anything that they could (*pause*)...

May: No, I couldn't.

Interviewer: You couldn't manage now?

May: No I couldn't, but yes, that's the thing that I miss the most, because they were old friends, sort of regular short nightly game.

Struggle

Struggle is part of life, and is not to be regarded as being negative. It is often through struggle that transcendence and subsequent spiritual growth occurs. Struggle, however, can take various forms and, according to where in the experience of struggle a person is, will depend on what hope they can see at that point. Christine refers to the time when she needed surgery, just after her husband had died, and she hoped that she would die then:

> **Christine:** I don't know what, I don't know that I'm really looking forward to anything. Um, no there are times I feel like I don't mind if I go to sleep and not wake up, I wouldn't know a thing about it, but that's the only way I'd like to go. I know we all have to go, but to when I don't know, um that lays ahead at this point in time, er when I had a clotted artery and a triple bypasses I really said 'Well Father I really hope you take me now, I don't want to come out', because that was when my husband had just died and I had to go straight in.

The following responses from participants' in-depth interviews, on the topic of hope, show the range held of a sense of hope, from no hope through to hope of eternal life. The responses were often influenced by earlier life experiences, and the tendency to continue to grow older in much the same way as they have been living for most of their lives. Roslyn responded in a similar way that many would do. She did not want to have to die slowly, over a period of time.

Roslyn: Just hope I drop dead if I do die.

Interviewer: What is it that gives you hope in life now?

Judith: I don't actually know, that's one subject that I have been puzzled about for many years. I have never yet delved into a situation where I know what will happen next.

Struggle is seen in Dianne's (MMSE 9) response to hope; her physical disabilities were obviously very difficult to deal with:

Interviewer: What gives you hope now?

Dianne: Hopes just to get away from this stuff. These legs and stuff.

Expectations of eternal life

Some spoke of life after death, as in the examples that follow:

Elvie: Well, just being as helpful as I can to people and/or going to heaven when I'm dead.

Interviewer: What do you look forward to?

Evelyn: Seeing Elsie again – that I get a spot in heaven.

Stella: What I look forward to is, what to, to be, what I am, not to be any longer, and what's got to be, to be and finished.

Interviewer: Mmm hmm.

Stella: That is all I ask, I don't want this, that or the other. And I look at it this way, I look out there and that, I have got a lot from there, and a lot from there. And I think the time will come, and well the thing is I say thank you God for what I had.

June: And now that is obviously that I am not altogether, you know, can't remember. But I, if, as long as my children, the two, and their things we are looking after, for doing it there, and everything going already for them, that's all.

Interviewer: What do you look forward to now in your life?

Tom: To die.

Interviewer: To die?

Tom: And I will have my life in heaven.

Miscellaneous foci of hope

There were other various foci of hope that were spoken of by the participants. For one man, Jim, catching a big fish was something he still hoped for. The variety of expressions of hope is seen in the range of responses from participants below.

> **Marilyn:** Oh, an interest in how the world's going, and what my friends are doing, and if they get married. You know I see them a lot, and they are busy asking me what I'm doing, I'm really trying to keep the house clean and do fascinating things like that when they come to tea, put them off forever.

> **Alice:** Still working.

People with advanced dementia are quite likely to take words literally. Note in the following that the interviewer paraphrased the sentence to get a response, and the response was certainly not what the interview had been attempting to elicit: hope was connected with 'getting out of bed in the morning'. Denise (MMSE 25) responded directly to the question – they need to make the bed, so of course you have to get out of bed.

> **Interviewer:** Yeah. What things give you hope now?
>
> **Denise:** Well I don't even think about such things.
>
> **Interviewer:** What makes you get out of bed in the morning?
>
> **Denise:** Got to get up.
>
> **Interviewer:** Someone tells you to?
>
> **Denise:** They come and they get me out of bed, they want to make the bed.

Another aspect of hope was associated with a moral perspective, of 'doing the right thing', as for Jill:

> **Jill:** Yes, that does not worry me at all, because I know that I am not stealing anything, or doing the wrong thing. I try to do the right thing, so that does not worry me.

Memories came into hope as well. Memories were a way of reinforcing hope, as for Jessica:

> **Jessica:** Remembering things.
>
> **Interviewer:** That gives you hope, remembering things?
>
> **Jessica:** Yes.

Interviewer: So you try and remember things?

Jessica: Keep playing them to retain them.

Fear

Fear is common among older people, and it is the opposite to hope. In fact, fear may be a strong emotion that blocks hope. This participant shows her lack of fear:

Interviewer: Is there anything that you are afraid of now? Any fears that you have?

Maureen: No I can't say (*pause*) trust in the Lord and that is all I can do.

Interviewer: As you mention the Lord, what kind of a God do you think he is, how do you see the Lord?

Maureen: Well, one thing, I always have him there, and I know he is looking after me, and it is in his hands what happens to me, that's all I can do.

Interviewer: And I guess you have, that goes a long way back in your life, that your relationship with God and your faith, and (*pause*)...

Maureen: Well, I always had, but I have more faith in him now than before because I am on my own and nobody near me all the time, on my own, but I have here, being looked after, and there is nothing more.

Fear was much less spoken of or acknowledged through questions for these people with dementia than it was for independent-living older people.

Strengthening hope among people with dementia

As can be seen, some of these people already had a strong sense of hope, but how can others be assisted to grow in hope? It is not as simple as saying that those who attend church will not be fearful, or will have hope. It is more than simply having a social activity that is protective against fear and hopelessness. For faith to be of assistance to the older person, it is a relationship and a sense of closeness with God that is protective. For Maureen in the excerpt above, it seems to be a simple faith, a simple belief, that gives her hope at this time. It is not about an intellectual connection with God, and, indeed, here hope remains for people with cognitive disabilities.

Summary

In both in-depth interviews and small group sessions these people with dementia did speak of hope, and of lack of hope. None of them appeared to be in despair, even those who said they had no hope. But it is possible, perhaps, that a person who was in despair would not have volunteered to be in this study.

Themes that they spoke of varied from a sense of acceptance of what lay ahead. Here it needs to be said that we cannot know whether having lost some degree of cognitive capacity would interfere with the acceptance of life that they were showing, and whether it might have been the same had they not developed dementia. At the other extreme, those who said they had no hope did not seem fearful of what lay ahead; in fact fear seemed to be mostly lacking among these participants. Again, that might be due to their diminished cognitive capacities. But then perhaps we could ask another question – do we people who are cognitively competent worry and fear too much? It would seem reasonable to consider that these people, like older people without dementia, were able to transcend the losses and disabilities of ageing, and move into 'being' from a 'doing' mode. There are examples of both in this chapter. However, the question of whether this move towards 'being' would need to have begun prior to the development of dementia cannot be answered from this study. It is only possible to say that there is evidence of participants who show signs of transcendence and hope in this study. Some participants noted the links between age and disability, for instance sight problems.

An important part of the participants' sense of hope came through memories of family, as so often in this study the need for connectedness and relationship was seen to be important. Even the memories of mothers and fathers, long dead, seemed to bring joy and hope to some of these people. These memories are a part of our life journeys, and the faulty memories of exact relationships, and the time of these, perhaps do not matter so much as the ability to hold them as part of one's identity. There was one participant who spoke of rehearsing these memories so that they would not slip away. Prayer and faith were important providers of hope for some: some waited to die and go to heaven; still others waited to be reunited with loved ones. This study was composed mainly of people from an Anglo-Celtic background, so Christians and people without a faith were the main participants.

10

Grief is Part of Life

Loss of relationship either through death or through geographical separation is closely tied to meaning in life. Meaning does not cease to exist because a person is dying; in fact, it is in facing death that it can be possible, perhaps for the first time, to see the meaning of one's life. Death was a topic in the long-running groups, and in fact, as might be expected, over a 24-week period of group sessions, of elderly and sometimes frail people, some participants were likely to die. This chapter addresses issues of dying, death and grief of these people with dementia.

Meaning in dying

Part of the small group process of spiritual reminiscence explored participant attitude and beliefs about dying and death. The topics were wide-ranging and covered aspects of grief that these participants remembered. As well, participants spoke of grief and loss in their individual in-depth interviews. An important distinction that we found between cognitively intact older people and those with dementia in this study was the relative ease with which more of those with dementia spoke about dying and death. They were more likely to name death as death, not 'passed away'. Grief seemed to be a normal topic among the participants, both in their small groups and individually. Fear of dying was not so marked, while it was a real fear for cognitively intact older people (MacKinlay 2006).

Talking about dying with the person with dementia and their families

Dying and death are not often topics raised with people who have dementia. Frequently, families feel uncomfortable in discussing issues of death and dying, both among themselves and certainly with those who have dementia. It is often said that the person with dementia will not remember, and it is distressing for them to be told about the death of loved ones, so why mention it in the first place?

As death and dying were subjects raised by group members and spoken about in the group settings, it is worth considering why we might be reluctant to talk about these issues with families and between staff and residents. One reason may be continuing taboos on these topics, and even a fear of death and dying, which is not only felt by residents, but also by staff and families. This may prevent families from broaching the subject, even when it is obvious that death may occur in the foreseeable future. One factor that may assist discussion of these topics is the setting up of advance directives, where the conversation may be facilitated between the person with dementia, families and staff.

We present material from the group sessions to demonstrate the type of conversations that these participants appeared comfortable to engage in. The participants were under no pressure to discuss these topics. The participants would sometimes seem to experience confusion of relationships, and seem often unable to name a particular relationship, yet connections with others were still important to them. This was obvious when, asked about where they found meaning in life, most said they found meaning through family. Relationship, or the term connectedness, which seems to express this better for those with dementia, was for these participants almost synonymous with meaning. Without relationship, without being able to connect with others, life has little meaning.

Speaking of death: Some examples from the study

Carol: Well, you see, a lot of people are, you know, frightened, or what else is the word, of dying, but we all have to go, so I just (*pause*)...

Rodney: A long time looking forward to the time when the Lord calls me. I know I am going to die; everybody will die, where the end will be. That I'll be ready when the Lord calls me, I should be satisfied, be able to say that the Lord has forgiven me, all off in debt.

Maureen: Well, I look forward to going to heaven, that's all I can say. I live from day to day, and that is about all I can say. I go to bed at night, I ask the Lord to look after me, I get up in the morning, I do the same, and that's all I can do.

Bronwyn: I look forward to the family being so close to me, and I know that I am prepared, everything has been arranged. And I thank the Lord for my family... I would like to say how happy I am that I live here and I can, if there was anything I could do to help anybody, anyone less fortunate than I, um, I'd try to.

If these people who have dementia can and do speak of dying and death, should those who do *not* have dementia also learn to speak of these topics? The findings from this study certainly show that death and dying are not topics off-limit for people with dementia. In fact, these people did not seem to show the same kind of fear of dying that many cognitively competent people show. This raises a number of questions related to fears of dying. Some would say that the perceived lack of fear expressed by those with dementia may be assumed to be because they do not know what they face. However, from the transcripts, it seems that this is doubtful, as will be shown in the examples used in this chapter. There may well be cognitive changes, but perhaps these allow the person to engage with topics that were not previously perceived to be suitable for discussion. One factor that seems to point to this is that cognitively intact people are often quite careful regarding what subject can be or can't be discussed, while people with cognitive impairments have a new freedom from these cognitive constraints. Fear itself can be paralysing and prevent people from dealing with difficult subjects. What is now needed are care providers who can meet people with dementia on their terms, and freely discuss topics that are on the minds and hearts of these people.

Grief as part of life

Most participants in this study described grief as being part of life. When asked about experiences of grief, Claire gave a response typical of others in the study, saying: 'Oh, when relations, you know, mother and father and husband and so forth, when they passed away, but they are the normal griefs and everyone has them. Nothing spectacular though.' Another participant remarked: 'I can't remember what it was. I've got a son and a daughter and they are kind to me and a husband who's very good to me.' The most important losses reported were loss of partner and loss of mother.

An aspect of grief that is worth considering with people who have dementia is the fact that, even though a person has died, there remains a relationship with the deceased person, albeit in a changed way. They still form part of the person's life, despite being physically absent (de Vries 2001). De Vries' work was with cognitively intact older people, but the same seemed to hold true for many of the participants in this study. Another loss that was spoken about was separation from children – and the experience of living in an aged care facility.

In response to the question 'Is there anything that you fear now, anything that you're fearful of?' Simone answered: 'I fear that I'll die alone.'

Facilitator: Yes, and there's that loneliness thing coming in again. Is that still a fear now that you're here in the hostel as well?

Simone: Well I think it's everybody's fear. I mean there's a quotation in the Bible that says: To seek first the kingdom of heaven, and all these things will be over unto you. Stand there beside you all the time, even though you can't see it, you can put your hand on it. I'm not a religious person. I'm err a lapsed Anglican, but err I was brought up in the Christian church when I was small. And I went to Sunday school 'cause you did what your parents told you in those days.

Another participant was asked: 'As you get closer to the end of your life, what do you look forward to?' Graham (MMSE 12) said: 'I look to seeing thee, my Jesus, I love thee, I know thou art my, feel the presence of sin I resign.'

These people with dementia, in the study, did not express fear of dying. They did not ask why 'God doesn't take me' as numbers of frail, but cognitively competent, older people had asked. What do these findings of lack of fear among people with dementia in this study mean? Is it that these people have moved to a place of peace and acceptance? Certainly, in their responses, most expressed a sense that *grief is part of life*. Do cognitively competent people have to work harder to overcome fears of dying? Or is it something different altogether?

Could it be that those who agreed to take part in the study were at peace, and we missed those who were distressed? Perhaps those who were distressed would not agree to take part in small group work. Gaining consent of those who do not wish to speak of dying is an important step to discovering the answers to these questions. It may be valuable to work on a one-on-one basis with people who have dementia, following the work of Faith Gibson (2004) on reminiscence. Gibson was able to find connections with the person's story, even when they seemed to struggle with language. Can we, through the process of spiritual reminiscence, help bring people who are distressed to peace and acceptance, as they face their dying?

Individual stories of grief and loss

Most of the examples are drawn from the individual in-depth interviews conducted prior to assigning the participants into small groups. The participants did more frequently speak about dying and death in their individual interviews than in the small groups. It is not clear whether this was the nature of the questions asked in the two settings, or whether it might be due to the presence of others, or even the attitudes of the small group facilitator. However, death was certainly a topic raised naturally in the groups as well as the in-depth interviews.

Acknowledging grief

In some groups the topic of grief emerged quite naturally through discussion, for instance in this group at week 16 of the sessions. By this time the group members knew each other well. This is a long excerpt, but valuable to follow through on the way the conversation about Stan's death was handled. Discussion of death and dying flows on to the fact that one of the members has an appointment with the hairdresser, and needs to leave the group at that point. At one point several of the group members were talking at the same time. The facilitator brings the focus back to Stan's death, acknowledging his death and supporting the group's members.

Facilitator: Are there any…we have had a bit of a hard week I think here haven't we, Mary?

Mary: In what way?

Facilitator: Well we have lost Stan this week. Did you remember? That he died on Sunday. And we don't have Joyce because today the funeral is on, and she has gone with her daughter. So there is some hard thing about living here isn't there?

Mary: Well I think it is a sad place to live, to stay, I do. You can't.

Facilitator: Is that because you are near the end of your life, and is that the reason do you think?

(*voices talking over each other*)

Mary: There are all old people here and there is something wrong with most of them. And you can never give them that venue.

(*Mary continues*)

Mary: No I get down sometimes, I am the biggest downer.

Facilitator: I wonder if I can get…would it help in that circumstance if when lost somebody, it doesn't matter how that would be, would it make it any easier if you knew that they were ready to die? How would you feel if you knew that personally? Wouldn't make it easier?

Mary: Oh no, you would miss them terribly. No I don't think it would make it any easier. It might at the time, you might think their time is up, but not really. You've got the rest of your life to live, you don't know when you're going to slip off. We've got to go I know that, I can't think of anything.

Facilitator: That's a big statement, that's nice, did you want to say anything about that, Mary?

Mary: No, not really.

Facilitator: Does it help when you lose somebody if you knew they were ready?

Mary: Oh yes it would, certainly would.

Facilitator: Would it make it any easier for whom, for you?

Mary: Might be, it would…I think the best thing of all would be to go suddenly.

Facilitator: Well I think that in Stan's case he did go suddenly didn't he? He was with us, suddenly he was gone. One day he was with us. You have got a hair appointment at eleven thirty, would you like to go through now? Because Kathy would take you now probably.

Mary: Well I suppose I better go.

Facilitator: Just as well we got you out of bed.

Mary: It is.

Facilitator: I won't be here, I am taking a holiday now.

Mary: I hope you have a very happy holiday.

Facilitator: Thank you, Mary, so nice of you. You go off to the hairdresser and we will see you when you get back, we will miss you. And then there was one. Bye, Mary.

Mary: I will see you again.

Margaret: Alright, Mary.

Facilitator: Bye, Mary. (*voices talking over each other*) Well just see how we go, it's ridiculous.

Margaret: It's just bad luck.

Facilitator: We had a guest you know, we couldn't tell she had a hair appointment. Even if we asked nobody would have been able to tell us. Okay, don't feel put on the spot now, Margaret. You can just say and you can stop whenever you want because it's quite a responsibility isn't it? And I do know that you quite like coming so that's lovely.

Margaret: What was I talking about?

Facilitator: We were just reflecting about having lost Stan so quickly.

Margaret: Oh, yes it's very sad for Joyce. They have been together for a long time.

Facilitator: And very often they used to recall how many years, and happy years, wonderful.

Grief is felt for little things too, such as not being able to cook any more, as well as for the deeper things in life, such as human relationships lost, as shown below:

Marjorie: All the wonderful things I used to do; I used to cook well, make cakes and things like that, and the children you see grow up and get married, and you and the husband just spend their lives. But B's [husband] gone to heaven.

Edith: Grief? Oh I had a little bit of sadness that way, but as I say you can't do anything about that either, you've got to put that behind, and just think quietly sometimes, sometimes.

May: I never think about dying. I mean we have got to go. We know that, but you don't dwell on it as you get older, I don't think.

Denise acknowledges her grief in a matter-of-fact way; there is sadness that she does not see her son more often, but as she said, 'so that's that'.

Often the participants spoke of the importance of the relationship with their own parents and their grief for them, even though they had been dead for many years. See both examples below.

Interviewer: Hmm. Hmm. Do you have any things that cause you grief over your life?

Denise: Well. Losing my husband, and my mother, 'cause I was very close to my mother and those are the things that caused me grief.

Interviewer: Hmm. Nothing with your children or...?

Denise: Ah no. Well my son of course, I don't see much of him at all, he lives in Sydney, and err disappointment more than grief.

Interviewer: Disappointment that you don't see him so often?

Denise: Yes. I would love to see them more often. Hmm, but I don't, so that's that!

Interviewer: Now are there any other um griefs that you haven't talked about yet?

John: Oh the normal ones with your parents, and err I don't think there's any. I've lost my daughter, I've lost my brother, not my daughter, lost my sister, that's right they just disappeared, sister and brother, they just died and that was that. And they were away from here, so the impact of it was not real great, and of course you said we had lost our son K.

Interviewer: Yes.

John: But other than that we've been pretty lucky.

Madeline acknowledged the main grief in her life, in the death of her husband:

Interviewer: What about grief in your life?

Madeline: Well, it was losing the family, you know.

Interviewer: Of course.

Madeline: Of course when I lost my husband, was the main thing.

Interviewer: Yes, that must have been hard then.

Madeline: Yeah. Because he has been dead now about four years, four or five years.

The continuing connection with those who have died (de Vries 2001) and who had been part of the significant relationships of participants is clearly seen in some of these examples, such as Christine speaking of her husband:

Christine: It is sad. Very sad, I never forget it, never. Occasionally I, something might happen and I'm and I'm by myself, I'll say 'Oh darling, you should have been here to hear that today', but er as he can't hear, he can't be here either, so there we are, but er no, but I think just the way they run this place is very, very good, and our [name] here is one of the main things I think that keeps people here, 'cause she's very kind…

Interviewer: Yeah, it's lovely.

Some participants stated that they did not have any grief in their lives, for instance Mary and Claire, who did not feel they grieved for anything. It is possible to ask whether they had forgotten the grief. It is interesting that there were such differences between the different participants in the study; for a large proportion of them, grief was very real, although mostly they seemed to handle it very practically, while still some others in the study, such as Mary and Claire, did not acknowledge any grief.

Difficulty in expressing grief associated with cognitive decline

Jill has a very low MMSE of 3. She struggled to express her grief, and then would forget what she was saying in mid-thought. For people like Jill, one-on-one interviews work best (the excerpt below is from her in-depth interview), as they are likely to lose their train of thought when surrounded by too many stimuli.

> **Interviewer:** Grief, yes, have you experienced much in the way of grief?

> **Jill:** I think everybody at some time or the other has had a little bit of grief, say they have been going to work, and then work (*pause*) for instance, I know, some people don't know. (*pause*) Ah. (*pause*) What was I saying?

> **Interviewer:** About grief.

> **Jill:** Oh, grief. Some people have grief when there is not really grief. If it is grief for those sort of people it is for themselves, it is not for everybody, and there is a difference, see?

> **Interviewer:** So have you experienced, what have been the biggest situations of grief that you have experienced?

> **Jill:** Death in the family, I felt grief, mostly. You have enough of your own, without broadcasting it, know what I mean, and then sometimes you have it, and you should not have it, it is none of your business, but you can't help that there is grief.

Getting a perspective on grief

Christine seems to have come to a realisation that she has choices – to let grief burden her, or to let it go. She has chosen to let it go and accept her situation.

> **Interviewer:** Do you have any griefs?

> **Christine:** Griefs. I don't think there's anything I could grieve about. I could feel sorry for myself when I don't see my family, but I don't grieve, 'cause the only person I'm hurting is myself. So I pick up and turn the telly on or do something else and put them right out.

> **Interviewer:** Yeah.

> **Christine:** Living here doesn't grieve me or anything like that, because there's nobody here that upsets you...if you want to be upset you could be, but no, my only grief is really not being near family.

The importance of animals for rural older people

Zilla was an older woman living in a rural community; her love of animals shone through in her life story.

Interviewer: Anything that you have grieved over?

Zilla: No, I don't think so. I grieve about the animals that died. Oh it was terrible, you know. I can't stand an animal dying, on me.

Finding meaning in grief

Death of a close family member is likely to be the cause of much grief, yet, as can be seen in the following excerpt, Bronwyn seeks to find meaning in their loss.

Bronwyn: And err we lost a son about 18 months ago.

Interviewer: Did you? Yes.

Bronwyn: With cancer.

Interviewer: Yes.

Bronwyn: And I realised that, um, that there must have been some purpose in it, just hard to find.

Interviewer: Yes.

Bronwyn: However.

Loss remembered from childhood

Loss of important relationships may be carried over many years. Sylvia remembered the death of her only brother, when she was about ten – how well she recalled the grief of her parents from that time. The significance for a family whose livelihood was tied to farming was devastating.

Sylvia: Or because the thing that comes to mind is that my only brother died when we was, ah, I think it was about ten year old.

Interviewer: Yes.

Sylvia: He had leukaemia.

Interviewer: Right, so that was a sad time?

Sylvia: It was very sad time and ah, um, for months, almost years I suppose, I remembered my mother and father both crying.

...

Sylvia: The brother that died was the only brother I had.

Interviewer: Yes.

Sylvia: And of course that was a tragedy for my father because he was depending on having a son to carry on the dairy work.

Interviewer: Of course, of course.

Sylvia: Not just the work, the whole family business.

Double grief: Loss of life partner and moving to residential care

Grief for the loss through death of a spouse of perhaps 40 or, these days, even 60 years has been said by some to be devastating. It would seem reasonable to assume that older people experience more episodes of grief than younger people, and to some extent they have had a lifetime of experiences of grief, beginning as young people; for example, moving house, changing schools, leaving school, loss of friends and pets and much more, all experienced as a normal part of life. But is this accumulation of grief much worse as it occurs in later life and includes the most significant losses of relationship, or have these older people, in some way, been prepared for the major losses of later life? It is not possible to minimise the experience of grief; it is a very personal and deep experience, and people tend to handle such experiences differently. Perhaps we might ask, how much grief can be experienced by one person? Some of the participants carried grief for both loss of a life partner and then being physically dislocated through needing to be admitted to an aged care facility following their partner's death. Sophie was one of those. In the initial meeting with her, it was difficult at first to get her to tell her story; the following excerpt from her in-depth interview illustrates her depression and her sense that there was no one who could help.

Interviewer: Where do you find meaning in life?

Sophie: Purpose?

Interviewer: Purpose. Do you feel that you are useless, or that life is useless?

Sophie: No, at the moment I am very depressed.

Interviewer: You are very depressed. Can you share with me a little bit just how you are feeling, because I think that would be important for us to...

Sophie: I don't want to be here, I don't belong here.

Interviewer: Okay. And have you been here very long?

Sophie: Three months.

Interviewer: Three months. And you are finding it hard to settle in?

Sophie: Yes.

Interviewer: Can you tell me a little bit about when you came in, what happened? Had you been living at home before?

Sophie: Well my husband died, passed away.

Interviewer: Your husband. So that was just before you came here?

Sophie: Yes.

Interviewer: Okay, so you are really still coming to terms with that, aren't you?

Sophie: Yes, very much.

Interviewer: Are you getting the kind of support to help you, or is there anything we can do to help you in that, have you got some kind of support?

Sophie: I don't know if anybody can help. Got to sort out myself.

Interviewer: Yeah. Have you got someone to talk to when you want?

Sophie: No I haven't.

This was an obvious situation where pastoral care would be recommended and of benefit. Spiritual assessment at admission would provide clues to Sophie's pastoral needs, with a plan for care being instituted at that time. Spiritual reminiscence may be a valuable means of assisting Sophie in her grief.

Overwhelming grief

While some may be able to accept grief and loss more readily, for some the experience can be overwhelming. Grief in dementia can be very hard. For some, cognitive levels make it hard for them to clearly express their grief, and yet the yearning for loved ones comes through as they speak; for instance, when the interviewer asked about the hardest things that this participant, Heather, experienced, she responded as below. Note that the relationship for Heather continues, even though it is apparent that Maurie, her partner, has died:

Interviewer: No, right now, for you with the hardest things, what are the hardest things for you now?

Heather: Yep, I feel more now, see I am not living with anybody now, you see I was living with Maurie, I feel a little bit more…it's harder for me.

Because I think I was leaning against a man. No I don't know, and I am telling you these things because you are both women. And uh, you know, it's a funny old world. My brother has been very good to me, brother, he is very good. And my dear old mum, I think she is still alive. And um, it's been hard, sweetie.

Interviewer: Yep.

Heather: But I still like to have a man somewhere, because I did not have a man, and I had Maurie, who was my dear Maurie, yes that's Maurie there. He was terribly good to me, good and kind to me. And he was a man, and I wanted a man, because my dad was not there any longer, you know. And that's sort of how it is, darling. And I could cry now and I don't want to cry for you.

Interviewer: You can cry any time.

Heather: My father died early, and one of the sad things, you know, he was older than she, and it was one of those things. And we were happy, and my husband to be, he was terribly good and kind to me. He would say that, c'mon, we would go somewhere, c'mon, and get your mother, and mostly your mother, my father had died, and we used to do a lot with Grandma, you know, do things, and we helped a lot, helped a lot, which is good. And I don't want to cry any more, sweetie. But don't, I don't mind crying if you don't cry.

Interviewer: I don't mind…we might cry together, who knows?

Heather: Funny things like that, and I did not think things could happen like that. Maurie came and picked me up today, you know, and took me out, you know, for a while, and I said, look you know, we have got to do something that we used to do. Instead of nothing, you have got to have something, you know, we have got to do something. But anyhow. Life goes on doesn't it?

Interviewer: It does, it does indeed.

Carrying family history and burden

Sometimes there were complex factors operating within families, for instance separation and rejection of certain members of the family that carried across the generations. This was so for Lotty. She seemed to struggle with the loss of family contacts, and her feelings for her mother, as Lotty felt her mother had cut her off from connections with particular family members. Lotty, however, made contact with these family members herself, which made her relationship with her mother probably even more difficult. She reflected on it here, in the excerpt below. For these older people with dementia, this time of life affords the only opportunity left for forgiveness and reconciliation. This is complicated due to the failing cognitive processes of these people. In some cases, it may be that healing for people like Lotty can come simply through being able to share their grief, even if loved ones are no longer alive for reconciliation to take place, face to face. What was open for Lotty was to work towards forgiving her mother. Lotty was able to rest in the knowledge that she had reached out to others to restore relationships and connections.

> **Interviewer:** Well, is there any grief that you still carry? What about the experiences of grief in your life, anything that you haven't managed yet?

> **Lotty:** Not really, because I didn't regret it, because um when my mother died I really, my feeling were, what a relief for her and relief for me, know what I mean? I did the best I could, and I knew I could do no more. But I'm afraid I never loved her very much, but she tried to do it to me as well, but I stuck with the family. We weren't allowed to the relations, well I, she did not want us to know our father's relations, but I was determined to do so and I did. I went against her will and kept in contact with them just on the surface. You understand?

Grief and faith

How important was faith in the experience of grief? On grief and faith, when the question 'Do you have any griefs?' was asked, Rose responded: 'No I don't have any regrets; I just sort it out with the Lord.' It is worth asking whether Rose associated grief with regrets; there is an association, although perhaps not a direct one, for cognitively intact people. For the person with dementia, it may be argued that the person may feel sadness for both regrets and loss associated with grief.

Elvie believed it was her religion that gave her support in her grief:

> **Elvie:** Yes, about I came out here for two years. I was going to stay two years and er met my husband and got married, and continued to work and work and I lived at…where did we, I forget the area. Ah it's beautiful there, but we only had a big shed, we built a shed and we never got any further, so put the windows in the end, but er…I suppose there's always grief when you lose somebody, but it's a natural part of living and dying.

> **Interviewer:** It is a natural part.

> **Elvie:** Yes. That's right. So I guess sort of we'll just go on as if I'm right. Some people here, there's one out there and she went berserk when her husband died and she's not right now, and I don't sort of feel that. They're still around.

Interviewer: You think spirits of people are around? So what do you think it is that's helped you actually work through your issues of, you know, of loss and grief in a way that you've been able to cope?

Elvie: My religion.

Having shared that, Elvie did not seem to want to share further; she had stated it clearly, and there it was. Elvie obviously had a depth of spirituality, as seen in her sense of the spirits being still around, and then her belief that it was her religion that supported her through grief. In the example below, Matt could see God's movement in what he and his partner had experienced in their lives and with their daughter.

Interviewer: Now as you look back over you life then, what about grief? Have there been big issues for you, occasions of grief in your life that you could name?

Matt: I think we had a surprisingly smooth life. Naturally you get periods where you're perhaps conscious of loss, grief, weakness. There have been minor, I would say minor, um, but it's not our doing, it's the Lord's opening doors, so much so, that afterwards when we came back our older daughter had to have a hip operation, and in fact she had another one later on and just recently she had her final one, and she's doing very well now and she's a senior architect in one of the big firms in Sydney.

Summary

Death and dying are topics that were discussed in both individual interviews and within the context of group sessions. Grief was a topic in the individual in-depth interviews done prior to assigning participants to groups. There was no hesitation among participants in talking about grief in these one-on-one sessions. In the group sessions, they were more likely to be discussed when group members and the facilitator had had a chance to get to know each other, although it was possible that the topics may have been raised earlier with experienced group facilitators. Participants seemed at ease in talking about these topics. Meaning, death, loss of relationship and need for connectedness could all be seen in the examples used in this chapter. We found spiritual reminiscence a valuable means of enabling the participants to speak of grief. In the small group sessions, group members were able to support each other, with the assistance of the facilitator.

11

A Theology of Dementia

Elizabeth MacKinlay

In a book on spiritual reminiscence and dementia, it is important to establish a context from which we can work theologically. This chapter focuses on a Christian understanding of the human person, and then of the person who has dementia. This starting point is an exploration of the nature of the person, created in the image of God. It is only after this exploration that we can move to understand a way into working pastorally, or for that matter, working in any of the disciplines that provide care for and journey with those who have dementia.

In fact, it is best to begin to explore a theology of dementia by looking at a theology of ageing, since dementia and ageing are so often linked together. What does it mean to be growing older? How does the ageing human being fit into this image of God that we will explore later in this chapter? Further still there are questions to be asked about the nature of the soul and its place in the person with dementia; after all, some people believe that only a shell of the person remains, or that it isn't the same person any more. For some, this view is extended to understand a loss of the 'self'. In this regard, Nancey Murphy (2006) argues strongly for the presence of a spirited body rather than a dualistic perspective that sees bodies and souls as different and separable. She writes that all that makes a human being:

> [s]hould be thought of primarily as that which provides the substrate for all of the personal attributes discussed (body, memory, character, moral perceptions and relationships): it is that which allows one to be recognized by others; that which bears one's memories; and whose capacities, emotional reactions, and perceptions have been shaped by one's moral actions and experience. (Murphy 2006, p.141)

This way of looking at the whole human being is a good place to begin to understand the importance of a unity of body, mind and soul, that will be of value in considering the person who has dementia. It is equally important, of course, to acknowledge the loved ones who make this journey with the person who has dementia, who may become care partners in this challenging journey. Keeping all this in mind, it seems best to begin with the nature of the person and their relationship with God and then return to the questions of the person who has dementia and theology.

Made in the image of God

The Abrahamic faiths hold that humans are made in the image of God; this is clearly set out in the Creation accounts in Scripture. We also know that at the end of the account of God's Creation in the book of Genesis, God declared that it was 'very good'. So we could assume perfection in all of creation. However, in contrast, the story of the fall begins with the journey of human sinfulness through disobedience to God. Does this mean that the range of perfect human beings, from then onward, was flawed? We may ask many questions about the nature of God's image in the human being and what it means. But in the Genesis account, genetic imperfections, and disease as well as death, arose at this critical point (the fall) that we recognise as pre-history. In Christian understanding, it is in the bringing in of the New Creation through the birth, life, death and resurrection of Jesus Christ that death is defeated and the whole creation that currently groans for renewal (Paul, Romans, chapter 8) will come into being. In the meantime, we live with imperfection, we live with diseases and mystery, grappling with questions that science alone cannot answer. It is in this context that we may consider dementia, but first I wish to explore what it means to be a person.

What does it mean to be a person?

To be a person, as I have already noted, is to be made in the image of God. What does that mean? It means to be endowed with the potential for relationship with God and others; it means to have creative potential; it means being able to take part in the life of the world, through work and play, through physical, cognitive, emotional and spiritual being. Image is not simply about surface things; for instance, when we say we are made in the image of God, it is not so much the physical nature of God but rather God's character that we are talking about. Humans, being made in God's image, are in a likeness to God. But what is this image of God like? Some years ago, when I was first working with older adults, one day, after I had spent well over an hour listening to the life story and spiritual journey of one woman, I asked her what she thought God was like; she paused and then, smiling, she said, 'Oh, God is all very Spirit, neither male nor female, but something greater than these.' What was even more remarkable about this woman and her statement was that as a small child she had thought that God was a severe judge who would punish her should she do anything wrong. This was an image of God that she had carried for many years of struggle and searching, and it was only in her late sixties that she was able to revise this image, and find the love and grace of God in her life. For her, the image of God was about relationship with God, at first distant and unapproachable; in later life this relationship changed as she drew nearer to the God she now saw with new eyes, something beyond her ability to fully describe, but having a sense of mystery and being beyond, and yet, at the same time, intimately present to her. Some will focus more on physical appearance and say that we know what God looks like because we have the memory of Jesus, God's Son, who lived among us. Still others will say that Jesus was simply a 'good man' and not God's Son. So there is great variety in the understandings of what it means to be made in God's image. Indeed, as in the story above, our human ideas of God can and do often change across our lifespan.

So far, I have written of human beings in the image of God, but what does it actually mean to be a *person*? This must be tied to human identity. What are the characteristics that are necessary for human identity? Murphy (2006) takes a philosophical view, arguing that to be identified as a person – and to be a person – means that there is continuity over time; it is necessary to consider the whole person – body, memory, consciousness and also moral character. Indeed, Murphy argues that human identity depends as much on character as it does on 'memory/consciousness and bodily continuity' (2006, p.138). Character will encompass the virtues and also emotions that make up the identity of the particular person. Thus Murphy (2005) clearly sets human identity in a theological context, and in so doing situates an emphasis on God's recognition, remembering and relating to each of us, which she notes will be essential to our post-resurrection identity. This effectively removes responsibility from us, as humans, to God for our afterlife.

God in relationship

To me, Jesus is the incarnate Son of God, both fully human and fully divine. So what does that tell us about God, and God's image? Very little, I suspect, unless we begin to unpack the relationship of God and his Son, and the Holy

Spirit. It is only then, once we begin to see God in Trinitarian terms as Father, Son and Holy Spirit, that we can begin to understand the nature of God. It is God-in-relationship that is so important in the context, not only of God, but also in the context of what it means to be human. It is *to* this Trinitarian God, *through* the Son *by* the Spirit, that we are held in relationship. This relationship of human with God is one of invitation and longing and loving on God's part, with our response being to simply accept God's invitation of relationship. This relationship with God is not an earned one, where we have been awarded a degree, or been appointed to a position of power and prestige, based on our merits. This relationship is one that is wholly based on God's love for us. It is not due to our great intellectual powers and abilities, our physical beauty or, indeed, anything that we can bring to win our way into God's love. God's love is so far beyond the imagination of human beings that it is in some ways almost impossible to comprehend.

So often as humans we look for relationships with others, either personal or in other spheres of our lives, such as our work, that will be earned and rewarded; God's love is not like that – it is free and unearned in any manner. We expect to be judged and found wanting, feeling that 'we are not good enough'. It is by grace that we are made right with God; that is the very nature of God, to continue to reach out to us in love. We find it difficult to know that God is like that. The exciting thing about this God who longs for a loving relationship with us is that it does not matter what our cognitive abilities are; nothing of our nature can make a difference, nothing can separate us from the love of God (Romans 8).

The Trinitarian nature of God and person in relation to Trinity

We are held in relationship with God, first through the once-for-all action of Jesus Christ – his death, resurrection and ascension. His action on the cross has meant that any separation between humans and God has been wiped away; has been abolished. This is a free gift to us. Our inability to live without sin, our inability to live without falling short of the glory of God, through our own will power, has been corrected. It has been corrected on our behalf by the work of Jesus on the cross. Thus we are bound in relationship, in mutual fellowship, with the Triune God, being one, of Father, Son and Holy Spirit. Moltmann (1991) wrote of the social doctrine of the Trinity, beginning with the biblical story of Christ and differentiating the Trinity and their means of fellowship: 'Jesus, the messianic Son; the Abba God, upon whom he calls; and the Holy Spirit. Who binds Jesus to the Father and through him comes into the world' (Moltmann 1991, p.131).

This was the first step in restoring the relationship between God and humans, and beginning the restoration of all creation. The incoming of the New Creation is Christ: 'behold, I make all things new' (Revelations 21:5). Even so, with our sins forgiven, we would still be alone in this world, without the Holy Spirit (the third person of the Trinity), who is our personal guide, advocate and counsellor, connecting us with God and the risen Christ.

It is God's initiative that establishes the relationship between God and the person. It is God-initiated, not human-initiated; therefore the person does not need to make the first move: we love God because God first loved us (1 John). Our response is to that initial invitation from God. Thus the person is first loved by God, restored to relationship through Christ and sustained in relationship by the Holy Spirit.

The soul and connections with God

Over the centuries, there have been different ways of understanding the concept of soul. Benner (1998) outlines a modern understanding of soul: 'The soul that was rediscovered was, therefore, not some ethereal, immortal, Platonic essence of being, but a very vital, embodied, spiritual core of personality' (p.12). Murphy (2005) takes this even further, noting that 'a physicalist anthropology (that is, a non-dualist account of human being) affects one's understanding of spiritual practices'. She explains that the biblical authors were not interested in

> cataloguing the metaphysical parts of a human being – body, soul, spirit, mind. Their interest was in relationships. The words that later Christians have translated with Greek philosophical terms and then understood as referring to parts of the self originally were used to designate aspects of human life. For example, *spirit* refers not to an immaterial something but to our capacity to be in relationship with God, to be moved by God's Spirit. (Murphy 2005, p.21)

Humans have long sought to identify that crucial component of being human that is the connection with the divine. For many, until the 20th century, this function has been assigned to the soul. In times of an increasing reductionist view coming from within the sciences and infiltrating the wider community, concepts of soul have become blurred and perhaps even meaningless to many people in the community. Is there a special part of the human being that connects with God? Or should we stop asking that question and ask, rather,

'How does God connect with humans?' Murphy (1999) seeks to explain the nature of human being in terms of physicalism and not in dualism, noting that this nature must be a non-reductionist physicalism. She concludes her arguments by denying a separate 'soul' within the human being:

> I want to suggest that religious experiences do not depend on any special facilities over and above ordinary human emotional and cognitive faculties. Their religiousness consists in (sometimes) their special content, but, more importantly, in their circumstances – circumstances that justify their being interpreted as acts of or encounters with the divine. In brief, religious experience supervenes on cognitive and/or affective experience in the context of an encounter with God. (p.568)

Thus Murphy is arguing for a very holistic concept of humanity. One part of the person is not split off from another; we do not have separate dimensions of the person – of the mind, the body and the soul. Rather, God works through human being and human becoming, connecting with persons in their bodily forms, as whole beings. After all, Jesus was incarnated into human flesh, and it is in this way that God connects with each of us, in our humanness, and that includes our bodies. Our emotional experiences and deepest senses of awe arise through our senses and are felt and expressed in our bodies. Green (2008) notes that examination of the Bible leaves 'no room' for 'segregating the human person into discrete, constitutive "parts", whether "bodily", or "spiritual" or "communal"' (Green 2008, p.49). In fact, humans are defined through their relationship to God, being like God, but different in that they are not divine. In the Genesis accounts (Genesis 1–2) there is no reference to humans being in possession of a separate 'soul'. In creation and in relation to the whole cosmos, humans are given the divine gift of life.

> Genesis does not define humanity in essentialist terms but in relational, as Yahweh's partner, and with emphasis on the communal, intersexual character of personhood, the quality of care the human family is to exercise with regard to creation as God's representative, the importance of the human modelling of the personal character of God, and the unassailable vocation of humans to reflect among themselves God's own character. (Green 2008, p.65)

Humans find true identity only in relation to God. Identity is always held within relationship; a person alone, without relationships, divine or human, cannot be affirmed of their identity in the absence of relationship. Murphy sums up the ideas of the person as an embodied spirit:

If we discard the concept of the soul as unnecessary, this is not to discard higher human capacities, but rather to open ourselves to wonder at the fact that creatures made out of the dust of the ground have been raised so high. What, indeed, is man that Thou are mindful of him? (Murphy 2006, p.146)

It is this embodied spirit in relation to others that is needed for human identity to be fulfilled. Identity is seen to be dependent not only on being an embodied spirit, but also for the embodied spirit to be part of the human community; to be in relation with others, and/or God. This is more readily understandable in considering the person who is cognitively competent. But what if the person has dementia? Does the person lose their personhood in the later processes of dementia? It is in this context that we may ask how identity can be worked out among those who have dementia. Is the person with dementia still an embodied spirit?

Identity: Recognising others. What of dementia?

Often we make judgements about the capacity of people with dementia to recognise others. If we assume that the person can no longer recognise others, it seems to provide a way of excusing cognitively competent people from continuing to interact with those deemed not to be able to recognise others. Christine Boden (1998) says that when she could not remember the names of her daughters, 'I still know who you are'; this is a different level of knowing. The knowing is there; however, the difficulty for the person with dementia may be that the exact naming of that relationship, or the ability to name that person, has gone. In other words, the label that we know them by has been lost. In a way, the identity of the person with dementia has been diminished by the lack of affirmation by others. Perhaps knowing and remembering are closely linked constructs, but not identical. Often others who do not have dementia will take this as an indication that the person no longer knows who the person is, or doesn't 'recognise' them, and this then becomes a justification for drawing away from the person, with the awful comment, often made in the presence of the person, 'She doesn't know who I am.' Maybe it is the expected facial expression that is missing, and the carer or visitor responds to this, without waiting, or exploring what is happening for the person with dementia.

An important component of identity is memory. Memory is more closely linked with cognitive capacity, and explains why it is such an important loss in dementia. But, even if memory is clouded, or lost, the idea of knowing may still be present. Perhaps it is something within the way the human functions that knowing may be connected with affective abilities, of which emotions and the spiritual dimension are a part.

The soul in dementia

Perhaps if we are able to see, with fresh eyes, that God has made us in his image, and that he communicates and connects with us in our wholeness of being human, not just as a body, mind or soul, this will bring a new sense of freedom for those with dementia. Like any other human beings, people who have dementia can still retain this sense of physicalism. In fact, it may be more appropriate to call humans embodied spirits. There is a wholeness in each person that is not diminished when cognitive abilities decline. Communication with other humans may become more complex, but communication from God does not depend on a certain minimum level of cognitive competence. There is a real sense in which this connection with God seems to be at the depths of our being, and our being is made up of all our human potential within each person. We found that in doing spiritual reminiscence with our small groups of people with dementia that their articulation of God in their lives was still real for them and they were able to talk about what God meant for them, even those with low MMSE scores. Bryden's (2005) writings of her experiences of living with her own early-onset dementia clearly show the importance of her relationship with God.

The person in dementia

So what does it mean to be a person who has dementia – in a theological perspective? Why is it important to explore this notion of personhood from a theological view? I think it is important because the theological view that you or I have of a person with dementia is going to colour the whole way and manner in which you or I approach this person. It will inform our values and beliefs about what is possible for this person. It will locate these beliefs and values firmly in how you or I think God regards the person with dementia. As a Christian, I am using a Christian perspective to explore this notion.

I first need to acknowledge the importance of my journey with Christine Bryden (Boden), and for her witness, as a person with dementia, that challenged me, and enabled me to make a huge attitudinal shift and look with new lenses at possibilities for people living with dementia (MacKinlay 2011). I needed to look at this disease through the lens of faith, and theology as well, to be able to be authentic to her as we shared this journey. By 2004, as she wrote her second book, she had reflected sufficiently on the question of who she would be when she died, to begin to provide some answers, both for herself and for others. This second book includes the story of her marriage since diagnosis with dementia. I have found her writing an inspirational part of this journey, with the struggle to know who she is, which is emerging, despite her cognitive decline. Christine wrote:

> At the centre of our being lies the true self, what identifies us to be truly human, truly unique, and truly the person we were born to be. This is our spiritual heart, the centre from which we draw meaning in this rush from birth to death, whenever we pause long enough to look beyond our cognition, through our clouded emotions into what lies within. (Bryden 2005, p.163)

It is from her whole being that she responds to life. Despite recent MRI evidence of the continuing progression of her frontotemporal dementia, Christine has continued to challenge the disease, and lives out the quote from her book (above).

Dementia is considered as both a biomedical disease and as a socially constructed disease. So to consider the person, made in the image of God, we need to consider both perspectives. At what point does the ageing human body begin to show signs of deterioration? It is important to realise that growing older is not a disease, although diseases can complicate the normal process of ageing. Is dementia to some extent part of the natural decay of the body and mind, such that St Paul wrote of in 2 Corinthians 4 and 5: 'we have this treasure in clay jars'. Paul refers to the human body, with all its weaknesses and impermanence, as the dwelling place of the Holy Spirit, given by God; the Holy Spirit that enlivens the person. Paul writes (2 Corinthians 4:16): 'Even though our outer nature is wasting away, our inner nature is being renewed day by day.' Further, he writes: 'For we know that if the earthly tent we live in is destroyed, we have a building from God' (2 Corinthians 5:1). Paul refers here to the fact that, even though our bodies may wear out, there is something else happening within the human being, something that is even mysterious; as the body wears out, so the spirit grows. Often Christians have held the body as being secondary to the spirit, and yet the honour in which the body is held is further highlighted in Paul's words on the New Creation (1 Corinthians 6:13): 'The body is not meant for fornication but for the Lord, and the Lord for the body.' Thus, from Paul's perspective, both body and soul are important. In fact we need to learn to see the person 'whole', not as separate compartments of being. Growing older in this perspective is not something to be feared, but something to be embraced. That is, of course, many would say, if we are cognitively competent.

In Paul's letter to the Ephesians, he sets out the relationship that God has prepared for humans, that 'just as he chose us in Christ before the foundation of the world to be holy and blameless before him in love, he destined us for adoption as his children through Jesus Christ' (Ephesians 1:4). This relationship is based on God's overwhelming love for us, which was set out from the very beginning of time. Being worthy in God's eyes has nothing to do with our worthiness. It is by God's grace alone. Paul can be said to be alluding to the affect with which we can know God (Ephesians 1:18) when he does not set out a means of knowing God by intellect, but by the heart: 'so that, with the eyes of your heart enlightened, you may know what is the hope to which he has called you'. This is a special way of knowing, but not by the brain; rather, it is an emotional or spiritual way in which we may know God. This allows for the inclusion of people with mental disabilities, including those with dementia. Even though the person with dementia may not show to us by words or facial expressions what they feel or know, this God of love will not abandon them.

Still a person?

So, does this all change with the onset of dementia? Is the person with dementia less of a person? How can we know God if we cannot remember? This is a fear expressed by numbers of people who have dementia and by their family members. In Western societies cognitive abilities, along with memory and autonomy, are highly prized. Dementia, which is largely identified by the losses of these abilities, is seen by some to leave the person stripped of so much that is deemed to be vital to be a *real* person. It is said by some that 'personhood' is robbed from the one who has dementia. For all the emphasis that has been given to personhood and person-centred care in recent times, in reality responses to people with dementia commonly treat them as 'sufferers' or, at best, as very limited beings. Our understandings of what it means to be a person are so tightly tied with 'doing' rather than 'being'; there is a sense that certain minimum levels of cognitive function are deemed essential to worthiness as a person. Therefore, people who have dementia do not qualify, or if they do, they are at least subject to a test of how much he/she remembers. For example, does he/she understand enough to attend a service of Holy Communion?

The part of memory in faith and community

Memory is not only an individual activity. Memory is part of a community being nurtured and supported in its faith. From the beginning, for the Jews, Muslims and Christians, memory and relationship with God has been central and provided the basis of support for the community of faith. The individual does not have to stand alone, but is situated within the community of believers. The sacred scriptures of each faith set out the story to be remembered.

In the Exodus, God instructs his people to remember, and to tell the story of the Exodus to their children down the generations. In the New Testament, Jesus says in the institution of the Last Supper: 'Eat this, drink this in remembrance of me...' Memory has a central part in the life of faith of the Abrahamic faiths, and this is rightly so. God has used human memory since the beginning to guide and lead and keep the story of which we are all members. Our lives and faith are bound in the remembrance of the story that is both God's and ours.

There is no mention of what happens if the individual cannot remember. But an important aspect is being part of a community of faith, and this community of faith supports and upholds the other members who may be in need. Paul draws attention to this when he writes of the church being the Body of Christ, illustrating the relationship of members as parts of the body, saying that the eye doesn't hear, nor the ear see, yet all parts of the body are necessary (1 Corinthians 12). Further, Paul wrote, the more lowly parts of the body are honoured by the stronger parts. Is it not like this with those who are disabled in some way, including those who cannot remember? As the Body of Christ, we are a community of faith that tends and cares for our weakest members. This does not mean that we take over what they can still do, but it does mean that we have a responsibility to walk with them, supporting and upholding them, finding out what they can still do, including them in this journey and affirming them as still being of value within the community. The term 'partners in care' fits this understanding of community.

We, in the Body of Christ, become the memory for the person who can no longer remember. The Bible gives clear guidance for the care of others, for example in visiting the sick and prisoners, clothing the naked and feeding the hungry (Matthew 25). Jesus spoke plainly of our duty towards others, and the story of the good Samaritan (Luke 10:25–37) leaves no doubt as to who our neighbours are and, further, what our duties to neighbours are.

What our duty to neighbour is not

In a society beset by secularity and rationalism, it is hard sometimes to stand outside the weight of media stories of the uselessness of older people and the burdens and problems of people who have dementia. A theology of the person in dementia is not a call to assisted suicide of those we deem not to be worth living. Nor is it a call to older people to end their own lives, so that *we* might have more to live on. Here we can return fruitfully to the basis of being human – being made in God's image; in this case there can be no point at which the life of a person is worthless. Still, in some communities and some aged care facilities, people with dementia are treated as though they are non-persons, simply objects to be fed or clothed, while their emotional and spiritual being is starved. In certain instances, staff and relatives still make judgements on the capacity of a person with dementia to 'know' or 'not know' something. We cannot know, ultimately, what another person knows or understands, unless they choose to or are able to tell us. The person with dementia, caught in the difficulty of communication, may 'know' but not be able to tell. Is it any wonder that 'behaviour' occurs at such times! Christine Bryden (Boden) at one time said that those of us who do not have dementia can be termed 'TABs', that is, 'temporarily advantaged brains', for we do not know when we too may lose our cognitive capacity, through accident, through a stroke or through dementia. The human person is far more than a cognitive being. I return to reflect that we are fearfully and wonderfully made (Psalm 139) – in the very image of God.

The self in dementia

What is this self that Christine Bryden (Boden) talks of? Numbers of people, including medical professionals, assert that the self is lost on this journey into dementia. Further, it has been asked, can a person with dementia think any rational thoughts at a time when their cognitive competence is declining – surely that is impossible? Christine was diagnosed first with Alzheimer's disease; about five to six years following her original diagnosis a revised diagnosis of frontotemporal dementia was made. A worker in health and ageing informed me that this just showed that Christine did not have Alzheimer's, and that the re-diagnosis discounted her witness to living positively with dementia. There is still confusion among some as to the terms used (types of dementia are discussed in detail in chapter 2). This lack of knowledge and subsequent attitudes are still unfortunately too common. Yet, many people who have worked closely with people who have dementia and many carers will tell anecdotes of profound statements and insights made by people who have dementia that seem to spring from nowhere. There is more to dementia than declining cognitive function. Christine's book *Dancing with Dementia* (Bryden 2005) shows what is possible in her continuing journey with this disease. She and her husband learn month by month, day by day, adjusting the steps of the dance to each other, continually learning and adjusting to changes in the disease, to live effectively with dementia.

It is said by some that, in dementia, the self ceases to exist. However, recent neurobiology findings do not reflect this position. Recent developments in knowledge in this field have allowed more thorough examination of the brain and its functions. Weaver (2004) writes of the damage done to the brain in dementia, and specifically dementia of the Alzheimer's type. He notes, importantly, that a person's knowledge of themselves, that is, the understanding that I have a 'self', lies in the knowledge that areas:

> thought to support the rudiments of experienced self-identity are outside of the brain regions most affected in the early and middle stages of Alzheimer's disease. Indeed, some, though not all, of these lower-level brain structures are resistant to the Alzheimer's disease process as long as the dementia patient is alive. (Weaver 2004, p.94)

Therefore, based on knowledge from neurobiology, it is possible that persons with dementia do retain a concept of self, well into the disease process, and to some extent until the late stages. This is an important understanding as it can overshadow perceptions of the person as no longer having a self, of being a vegetable. It provides a basis for what numbers of those caring for people with dementia have been saying for a very long time: the person remains, the self remains, even in the midst of changes and cognitive deterioration.

The need for community in dementia

I have written about the significance of relationship and the Trinitarian perspective on God-with-us. A practical outworking of this is seen in Christine Bryden's words as she contemplated her future journey into dementia:

> As I travel towards the dissolution of my self, my personality, my very 'essence', my relationship with God needs increasing support from you, my other in the body of Christ. Don't abandon me at any stage, for the Holy Spirit connects us. It links our souls, our spirits – not our minds or brains. I need you to minister to me, to sing with me, pray with me, to be my memory for me. (Bryden and MacKinlay 2002, p.74)

Although we may argue that we don't have a separate 'soul', if we take a holistic view in considering the person with dementia, it can easily be seen that the community, and in this case the community of faith, can play a crucial supportive role. The person with dementia may be held by the community, by supporting the memories of faith, the Scriptures, the Eucharist, prayer and the familiar patterns of worship.

Christine's words echo the thoughts of Balthasar (in McIntosh 1998, p.113) that 'all human consciousness is irreducibly interpersonal, that is, I am aware of myself and of anything at all because "I" have been addressed by another'. Further, McIntosh (1998, p.113) notes:

> ...the patterns I come to 'know' anything at all are ultimately congruent with the trinitarian relations of infinitely giving love. This means I will only know insofar as I am ready to love the other, learning in other words to know as God knows Godself.

If this is so, it has important implications for our relationships with people who have dementia. Human beings do not exist in a vacuum, in isolation, yet sometimes by the way that dementia is defined in the biomedical paradigm this would seem to be the case. The person with dementia is asked to stand apart from other humans and 'prove' that they are a rational being. If we have love one for another (John 13:35) then we can be enabled to love the one with dementia. The need for interpersonal relationship, both with God and others, of those with dementia, is like the need for interpersonal relationship with other human beings; it is simply part of being human. It is human fear of mental illness that drives the stigma of dementia and causes us to feel separate from the person with dementia.

Resting in God's love and grace

Does a person who lets go of the need to control and gives over control of their life to God experience dementia differently from one who tries to retain control for as long as possible? For Tyndale (Werrell 2006), this depended on a relationship that is worked out by God, not the person, in that it is by God's love and grace alone that the person is right with God. In this condition, the person has no need to strive to retain control, nor are they 'out of control'; they are, rather, within God's loving care. Giving control to God is not a passive way of being, in which the person is a mere puppet. Walking in God's will involves being all that God has called us to be, physically, emotionally and spiritually. It is growing into Christ, the very image of God. The person with dementia can be caught up in the community of faith that holds and supports memory and the very essence of the person.

Summary

I have argued in this chapter for an understanding of the person, made in the image of God, a perspective from which we can continue to honour and support the person, even as their cognitive abilities decline in dementia. I have argued for the importance of community, especially the community of faith in which identity is upheld. But I also acknowledge that personhood can be affirmed and upheld within caring communities outside of faith communities. It is how we value the person who has mental disabilities that is important, and hence how we care for the weak and vulnerable.

There are different ways of understanding the person with dementia. The way we choose to understand the person with dementia will be crucial to the care that is available to these people and – can I go further? – crucial to the well-being of society. Should the view of the value of the person – made in the image of God be eroded by the knowledge and values of secular societies, then there will be little hope for people with dementia. Already in some quarters, there are calls for assisted suicide or even euthanasia of people who have diagnoses of dementia.

We are at a critical time in history in Western societies, where materialism and rationalism seem to gain importance above values that may be hidden, in humility, love, joy, forgiveness, hope and reconciliation. Where productivity becomes the only goal of humanity, we, like the Nazis, will become an abhorrent society, doomed to failure and oblivion.

PART 3

Practice of Spiritual Reminiscence

12

Maximising Effective Communication

At the core of spiritual reminiscence are the questions: How can we communicate effectively with people with dementia in a way that increases our understanding of their experience? How can we use this information to enhance their quality of life? How can this process of spiritual reminiscence assist these people to find meaning in the face of dementia? Facilitating spiritual reminiscence groups requires good communication skills and the ability to help those with dementia express their thoughts. It means allowing time, watching carefully for non-verbal interactions and using thoughtful questioning. Many authors contend that good communication skills from carers are the key to enhancing physical, psychological and spiritual care (Bird 2002; Goldsmith 1996; Herman and Williams 2009; Killick and Allen 2001; Kitwood 1993; Naue and Kroll 2008; Smith and Buckwalter 2005). Using spiritual reminiscence is a way to encourage and enhance this communication.

This chapter examines the communication and facilitation issues that impacted on the spiritual reminiscence groups. Each facilitator faced many challenges when leading the groups. Some of the participants had hearing difficulties and were better placed near the facilitator. Some participants tended to dominate the conversation and the facilitator had to ensure that other participants also had a say. As in the other chapters, you need to keep in mind that these participants have dementia – some of the interactions are very insightful and demonstrate how those with dementia can engage in a discussion. These responses are very valuable as there are few studies that consider the perspective of the person with dementia life and how they are coping with dementia.

Why use small groups for spiritual reminiscence?

All participants in the spiritual reminiscence project had an individual interview before participating in the small groups. On an individual basis, most of the participants were able to give thoughtful responses to the issues of spiritual reminiscence. However, one of the aims of the project was to give those with dementia the opportunity to experience the benefits of being part of a small group over a longer period of time and thus increase the connectedness between participants. The role of the facilitator was to use communication strategies to encourage interaction between the facilitator and participants and among participants. In fact, this type of therapeutic communication may affect both the quality of life and quality of care in aged care settings (Levy-Storms 2008). Older people with dementia in residential care seem to speak to each other infrequently. One study identified that nearly half of all aged care residents never talk to their roommate because of speech or hearing impediments (Kovach and Robinson 1996). Although we often see groups of people with dementia sitting together, frequently there is little or no communication between them. In fact, even in activity groups, most communication is between the person leading the group and individual group members. In the spiritual reminiscence groups, especially the 24-week groups, it was often noted how individuals conversed among themselves, enhancing ongoing interactions.

Group size and length of sessions

Participants were allocated into either a short six-week group or a longer 24-week group. The decision on which type of group the participant joined was based on a number of factors. First, participants were allocated to shorter groups if their level of dementia was greater, based on the MMSE. It was felt that small (between three and four participants), shorter groups would suit those with more cognitive difficulties. Participants with a higher MMSE tended to be allocated to a longer, slightly larger (four or five participants) group. Second, the ability of the facilitator to continue a long group for 24 weeks was taken into consideration. Frequently issues of staff changeover, and the ability to provide continuity of group sessions over the longer term, impacted on the length of the group. Finally, allocation was for convenience. Some facilitators managed two groups at once – one long group and two consecutive short groups of participants. Overall, however, the participants who seemed to develop the most lasting relationships were in the longer groups.

Facilitating spiritual reminiscence groups required considerable commitment from the facilitator and the aged care facility. The timing of the groups needed to ensure that other activities were not interrupted and that the facilitator also had the time to manage the group. In one facility, the 24-week group also coincided with a major building programme that necessitated much building noise and even the transfer of some participants to another facility. Groups also had to function alongside visits from relatives, friends or doctors.

Because of the nature of dementia it was sometimes found that participants were not able to be included in the reminiscence groups. The role of the facilitator was to identify those for whom the group process was not suitable. As a result, some participants were excluded. In one group, a couple of the participants found it very difficult to sit in one place for an extended length of time and contribute to the group. This resulted in one of the facilitators following a participant, asking questions and attempting to record answers – this did not contribute to the group process at all and the participant was excluded. In another group, one participant with word preservation continually interrupted and was unable to join in the discussion with the rest of the group. Again, she was excluded from the group. Both of these participants were interviewed individually at the start of the study.

Communication challenges for those with dementia

People with dementia have some specific communication challenges. All participants in the project had a diagnosis of dementia, but the types of dementia were not necessarily specified. Different types of dementia result in differing types of speech, communication and understanding. These include severe anomia (impaired recall of words), comprehension deficits and impaired object recognition (Croot *et al.* 2009). In addition to those issues related to dementia, participants also experienced the usual age-related problems of hearing loss. Age-related hearing loss is one of the most frequent ageing changes in the older population. In Australia, up to 74 per cent of people over the age of 70 years have hearing loss (Access Economics 2006). Figures are similar in the UK (Allen *et al.* 2003). Older adults with hearing loss have a lower physical and mental health status (Hogan *et al.* 2009) than those with no hearing impairment. It makes those with deafness particularly vulnerable in aged care, as they are less likely to interact socially and join in facility activities. People with both dementia and hearing loss are significantly disadvantaged in relation to communication. Mabel put this very nicely into her own words:

Mabel: It's hard sometimes to express what you feel, 'cause you just can't find the right words, and you feel that you sound a bit stupid if you say what you're thinking, you know.

Kitwood (1997) wrote that communication is the responsibility of those *without* dementia, that is, we should not expect the person with dementia to meet our expectations for communication. Those with dementia often have difficulty expressing themselves. They may have trouble finding the right word, beginning an interaction, concentrating on questions and remarks and ending an interaction. Unlike conversation with cognitively intact people, which can assume a pre-set form, conversation with those with dementia needs special properties on the part of the receiver. Kitwood (1993) provides the analogy of tennis when trying to emphasise this communication. A tennis coach can return any ball hit by a novice, whether or not these shots meet the requirements for a tennis game – the coach can help the novice to keep the rally going but the coach is not aiming to win the game. This is a valuable analogy – the role of the carer or facilitator or family member is to keep the communication going, even if it seems the conversation is off track or not meeting expectations. This communication needs much skill and will often be creative and demanding but intensely satisfying.

Having communication difficulties does not mean that those with dementia have less to say or that what they say is not meaningful. Work by Goldsmith (1996) and Killick and Allen (2001) demonstrates that those with dementia not only can contribute to meaningful conversations but also have plenty to say. Frequently communication with those with dementia is superficial, trivial and patronising. Little emphasis is given to meaningful questions that allow the older person to pose considered answers about things that interest them. This comes about for a number of reasons, including lack of time on the part of staff, feeling ill-equipped to deal with the responses and thinking that the person would be unable to communicate adequately to respond. There are many examples in the literature demonstrating poor communication between carers and residents. Part of the stigma associated with dementia is the commonly held view that meaningful conversation cannot occur – so it is not tried. We accord an individual the status of a person when we acknowledge his/her uniqueness and value. At the heart of a person-centred approach there is an emphasis on a relationship in which there is the capacity for each person to discover something new, creative and nurturing in another person (Goldsmith 2001). Kitwood (1997) describes this as the ability to be present for the person with dementia. It entails letting go of the constant *doing* involved in dementia care and become involved in *being* with the person. Good communication reinforces the notions of person-centred care.

There are a number of common communication difficulties experienced by those with dementia. In the small groups, frequent references were made to the problems they experienced – not only to memory issues but also communication issues. It is interesting to see that participants showed considerable insight when discussing some of these problems – again, something we do not always expect.

Word finding was mentioned in a number of groups. Participants described the frustration they experienced. They referred to this in a number of different ways, but all were aware of this as a progressive loss due to their increasing dementia. Beverley sums this up neatly by saying that her brain 'can be shut'.

> **Beverley:** What I worry about? What do I worry about? I can't think of anything special.
>
> **Interviewer:** You were talking earlier about not finding the right words, does that ever worry you?
>
> **Beverley:** Oh yes. My brain can be shut.

The following excerpt gives another example of the ways that participants described their difficulties with communication. Jennifer talks about not being as free with speech:

> **Interviewer:** Is there a sense that you have a sense of purpose in your life?
>
> **Jennifer:** Oh no, I, oh, I don't know what I wanted to say.
>
> **Interviewer:** Okay, just take your time.
>
> **Jennifer:** I am not remembering things as I used to.
>
> **Interviewer:** Right, is that a concern for you?
>
> **Jennifer:** Pardon?
>
> **Interviewer:** Is that a concern for you?
>
> **Jennifer:** Well, I don't seem to be as free as I was. What do you want to know?

In the following excerpt Ben and Anita are trying to explain how they feel about their memory loss. They talk about this in response to the question of how they feel about getting older. Despite their dementia they are able to communicate if there is time allocated, and the facilitator helps with understanding.

Facilitator: How do feel about getting older?

Ben: Hardly say enjoyed, but...

Facilitator: Managing to adapt to it are you?

Ben: Managing to adapt to it. Except for memory losses.

Facilitator: Yes, that must be hard to come to grips with – is it?

Ben: Yes.

Facilitator: How does it affect you?

Ben: Just kind of frustrating.

Facilitator: So, I remember you saying something to me this morning, you wanted to tell me something, you got half way through it and then you couldn't remember the next word. Do you find that that's the frustrating part?

Ben: Yes, that's the frustrating part.

Facilitator: So you know what you want to say in your mind, but sometimes when you go to say it, it won't come. Is that what happens?

Ben: I just black out.

Facilitator: Right. Do you find that, Anita, does that happen to you sometimes?

Anita: I find that I just can't think when I want to say.

Facilitator: Yes, you know there's something that you want to say. You go to say it and it is gone, or you just can't express it.

Anita: Won't, can't speak it.

Facilitator: It won't come out.

Anita: Yes.

Facilitator: But in your mind you know what you want to say.

Anita: Yes, I suppose I do. I've been going to ask, Doctor, what's the matter with me? You know...

Maureen, in the following excerpt, is responding to some comments made by the facilitator. It is the last week of a six-week group and Maureen is expressing her thanks for the opportunity of the group.

Maureen: Well I think you have understood, and that helps, what I have. Just that I wanted to be able to express what comes into my brain doesn't come easily to express the way I want it to be expressed.

People with dementia are in danger of losing their identity because that identity rests on appropriate responses from other people. By not responding to, or by ignoring or belittling, the person's stories, we are implying that they have no value. David Snowden describes an amusing incident when an older man with dementia, who had almost ceased to speak to his wife, was very talkative when asked about his 'feelings' in a study interview: 'Imagine his wife's surprise when she suddenly heard her husband's voice from the other room. One of the things he said to the researcher: "I don't talk anymore because no-one listens anymore"' (Snowden 2002, p.195).

Sometimes when we first met with people who had dementia, and asked them if they would share some of their life story with us, they were reluctant as they thought their story was not important. One participant replied: 'But I don't have a story to tell, I'm only an ordinary person.' Yet, when we took time to sit with them and affirm them as people worth listening to, the story would emerge, gradually and confidently. When you listen to another person you are acknowledging them as an individual in their own right. This has been noted in hospital wards where nurses spend far less time interacting with patients with dementia because it is felt that they cannot understand and therefore cannot interact (Ekman *et al.* 1991). If you receive no response to your story, then, after a while, you stop trying to participate or contribute to a conversation.

Elderspeak

We know that 'elderspeak' is commonly used in residential aged care. The term elderspeak has been coined to express the patronising style of speaking that is sometimes used with older people; it includes raising the tone of voice, speaking down to them as though older people have little ability to understand, using a plural pronoun (are *we* ready for *our* bath) and inappropriate terms of endearment (Williams *et al.* 2009). It also tends to be the way we speak to children, so we are immediately showing no respect to the older person – it indicates that we do not think the person is competent. Using elderspeak with an older person implies that we think they are incompetent and have poor memory skills. Those on the receiving end of elderspeak have their own negative stereotypes reinforced, thus eroding self-esteem and the person's evaluation of their capabilities.

In a study examining elderspeak as a communication style, it was found that elderspeak predominated and normal adult conversation was infrequent. This study found that there was an increase in behaviour problems and resisting care with both elderspeak and silence during care episodes (Herman and Williams 2009). Other studies have found that elderspeak encourages increased dependency, especially in residential care settings (Williams *et al.* 2009).

Finding meaning

When we planned the spiritual reminiscence sessions, many carers asked whether we were realistic in thinking that older people with dementia could respond to the questions we were intending to ask. It was difficult for them to imagine that people with dementia could respond to these topics related to meaning – yet, as we found, most participants responded very well and enjoyed the opportunity to engage in meaningful communication on an equal footing.

However, not all participants found it easy to engage with the process. We found that Janet was challenging to draw out into conversation. Notice that the interviewer in the example below tries to use every possible cue from what Janet has of her photos and so forth in her room. The interviewer also allows long pauses of silence, in case Janet may respond, but there was very little forthcoming. This would have been one of the most difficult interviews, as mostly participants seemed to warm to the interview process and participate readily, even if unsure initially. Notice that factual questions do not seem to help these people to respond. This was an early interview, and we would hesitate these days to ask questions that require concrete answers, as we have found that, where a participant has trouble speaking, asking for facts increases their anxiety, and they are less likely to be able to respond. It is important to stay with 'meaning' questions.

> **Interviewer:** So, Janet, what can you tell me have been the really good things, what have been the good things in your life up to now?
>
> (*silence*)
>
> **Janet:** Um, well (*pause*) what do you mean by telling you?
>
> **Interviewer:** What have been the good things that have been in your life, what have been the fun things that you have enjoyed the most?
>
> **Janet:** Oh, that is a hard thing to say, isn't it?
>
> **Interviewer:** Yes, yes.

(*silence*)

Interviewer: What have been some of the things you look back on with joy? Have you got a, had a family, have you done lots of things in your life?

Janet: Oh yes, yes, yes. I had a family.

Interviewer: Yes, how many children did you have?

Janet: Um.

(*silence*)

Interviewer: Can you remember how many children? Did you have any sons and daughters?

Janet: Well, I, hmm.

Interviewer: Who is this photo of?

Janet: I (*pause*)...

Interviewer: That's you in the middle, isn't it?

(*silence*)

Interviewer: Who is that? Do you know who that is?

(*silence*)

Janet: Well that is my, um, (*pause*) Susan and her mother.

Interviewer: Is that one of your granddaughters?

Janet: Yes.

Interviewer: Yes. Is that a granddaughter as well?

Janet: Yes.

Interviewer: Looks lovely. And who is this in this [photo]?

Janet: You want me to tell (*pause*) that's myself.

Interviewer: That's you is it? And who is that? Is that your husband? Would that be your husband?

Janet: Yes, I think so.

Interviewer: Hmmm. And what things have made you happy?

Janet: Oh. (*silence*) Oh I think I have some, going home to my daughter's place and that sort of thing.

Interviewer: Yep, and that is always a happy occasion is it?

Janet: Oh yes.

Interviewer: Yes. I see you have just had a birthday. You have got some birthday cards up there.

Janet: Yes.

Once Janet was in the group she responded to direct questions but did not offer any additional information. She predominantly answered either yes or no to questions and comments. She was in a small group that also had one of her particular friends in it – so she was surrounded by people she was familiar with. The following is an exceptional response:

Facilitator: What are, or have been, the best things about relationships in your life?

Janet: Remembering to make friends.

In another interaction she responded to a question about whether she participated in any of the religious activities in the residential home. Again, we get a glimpse of 'Janet' – we need to listen for the words and not simply dismiss the conversation if there is no immediate response.

Interviewer: You do? Okay. How important is it to you? This Bible reading that you take part in?

Janet: Oh well I actually prefer a book.

The following is from the initial interview with Jim. During the interview he spoke of his pleasure in fishing – when asked about any troubles he responded as follows:

Interviewer: Do you worry about any things now?

Jim: Yeah. Ah I forget them as soon as I catch them.

Interviewer: Oh right, yeah.

Jim: 'Cause I'm generally bang, let them go again, see? That's all I used to do.

Interviewer: When you had a worry you took care of it quickly did you?

Jim: Yeah, I'd just go and seek the best section.

Killick and Allen (2001) suggest that in order to make meanings from words that do not seem to offer an immediate response to a question or comment, there is the need to bring to the interpretation 'an imaginative openness' that can help us to understand – rather than dismissing the response as nonsense.

Non-verbal interaction

When it becomes more difficult to speak or to express yourself using words, non-verbal behaviours become very important. In the groups, people helped each other and used non-verbal interactions such as touch and leaning forward to reinforce the relationships in the groups. Hubbard *et al.* (2002), in their study of non-verbal behaviours, found that these interactions were very important as part of the social interactions of people with dementia. They found that non-verbal behaviours were used to initiate, enhance and maintain conversations, to amplify interactions, to describe situations they could not find words for or to draw attention quietly to personal needs.

Prior to each spiritual reminiscence session the research assistant would help to gather everyone together and take them to the allocated room. During the session the research assistant would observe all the interactions that took place between participants and the facilitator. The following is from one of the journals. It is week 4 of a 24-week group. This group developed supportive relationships quickly. One of the participants (Bob) had missed two weeks, but the group remembered him and welcomed him back. Another was quite hard of hearing, but the facilitator and other participants made sure that she was included. In this excerpt, another participant repeats comments or attracts her attention when it looks as if she has missed something:

> Good interaction between the participants. All participants look at the person who is speaking, laugh and respond appropriately. Bob seemed to fit back into the group with no disruption.

> Maude has difficulty hearing and sometimes misses out on the discussion. However, the Facilitator tries to include her by sitting next to her each session, and repeating comments or questions for her when it appears she hasn't heard them. It was evident that Alice was making sure to include Maude in the discussion when she leaned over, tapped her on the arm and repeated a comment for her.

Even relatively early in the life of the group participants are helping each other. The journal goes on to record many such instances of participants helping each other. The following excerpt was written at the end of one of the six-week groups. Even over this short period the research assistant noted differences in the interactions between participants.

> I noticed over the 6 sessions that the participants became relaxed and open with each other quite quickly, interacting well – changing from closed body language and short responses to relaxed, open body language,

talking and laughing. It seemed to have a positive effect on them in terms of interacting with others, being relaxed and laughing, for at least a short time after each session ended. However, as observed, when back with the other residents, the participant's openness and talkativeness tended to subside again.

The research assistant in this excerpt noted how, once the groups had completed, participants went into the communal area and were initiating conversations with other residents. However, after receiving no encouragement to continue this interaction, they again became silent. If this engagement could be encouraged to continue, it could certainly change the verbal and social interactions between people with dementia. These interactions are possible, but require nurturing and encouragement.

Ways of effectively facilitating the group process

As Kitwood (1997) has said, the responsibility for good communication rests with those who do not have dementia – in this case, the group facilitators. The group facilitators were essential to the success of this project. To assist facilitators, a training session was held prior to the commencement of the groups. One of the first tasks was to identify some of the differences between a 'group leader' and facilitator. Whereas a group leader might lead and direct a group, a facilitator guides, supports and affirms the work of the group. The role of the facilitator is to tune in to the needs of the group and identify ways to bring out the best from each member of the group. It is important that the facilitator allows time for the group members to share, is respectful of each person's contribution and encourages quieter group members to contribute to the conversations. The facilitator also needs to be aware of body language and pick up on other non-verbal cues.

The group time is for the group members to share, not for entertainment by the facilitator. The skilled facilitator draws the participants into deeper sharing while at the same time maintaining a level of comfort within the group. The facilitator should always listen to the participants and be ready, if needed, to reflect back to clarify issues and be guided by the needs of the participants. There were specific questions associated with each week of the group process, but the facilitators most in tune with the group's needs used these as a guide and an invitation to participate rather than being prescriptive. Allowing participants to set the pace and guide the discussion provided the most meaningful responses.

Group facilitators who were able to encourage the most group responses asked one question at a time and gave the group members time for thinking, processing and responding to questions, taking account of the added time that it takes for a person with cognitive difficulties to respond to questions. In recent unpublished research we have found that it sometimes takes 5–6 seconds after a question for the person with dementia to be able to respond, far longer than for people without cognitive deficits. It is important to realise that the person may well be able to indicate their wants and needs, given sufficient time and support to await an unhurried reply. The following example demonstrates some of the issues when there is not enough time given for participants to respond. It is interesting to note that another participant (Hetty) recognised that Louise needed more thinking time.

Facilitator: What do you worry about, Louise?

Louise: Oh I don't really.

Facilitator: Favourite worries?

Louise: No I don't.

Facilitator: What do you think about most of the time?

Louise: Oh I don't know, I don't know.

Hetty: She has no time to think.

Facilitator: No time to think.

Giving time for a response will often mean allowing silence to occur. In group work, the role of the facilitator is to understand when silence is needed and allow this to happen and not feel embarrassed by the silence. Silence is a powerful tool in communication. It is not a concept found frequently in aged care. Just sit quietly for a minute and listen to the background noise all around. Paradoxically, however, for the majority of the time, older people with dementia are sitting quietly and not interacting with anyone. When we speak to people who are being 'too quiet' in response, we often want to fill up the space. Just because a person is quiet in response to a question does not mean that they are unable to answer. Often time needs to be given to formulate an answer – continuing to ask questions or make comments, as in the interaction between the facilitator, Louise and Hetty above, does not allow thinking time, as Hetty notes. To allow silence we first have to stop talking!

We speak to fill up gaps for a number of reasons. It is sometimes uncomfortable to be silent; we may think the other person has not understood what we have said or is ignoring us. Killick and Allen (2001, p.163) cite

Starkman (1993), who contends that we need to 'learn to sit in the silence'. Personal care, however, carried out in silence, can increase the instances of 'problem behaviour' – there is a time and a place for silence (Herman and Williams 2009).

The role of the group facilitator

The communication strategies demonstrated by the facilitator could 'make or break' a group. When listening to the recordings of spiritual reminiscence groups it was interesting to note how much the difference between responses depended on the group facilitator's style. Prior to the commencement of the project in each facility, the group facilitators had training in techniques to enhance their communication and group facilitation skills. The research assistant present at all the group sessions was of considerable assistance in assisting with challenging communication issues and in debriefing the facilitator at the completion of each session. It was good if the facilitator had had the experience of being a participant in a spiritual reminiscence session, prior to facilitating a group themselves.

The facilitator had to be very comfortable with the notion of personhood and be able to identify the behaviours that led to 'malignant social psychology' (Kitwood 1997). In addition, s/he needed to have a good understanding of the elements of behaviour that encourage person-centred care and also the guidelines for managing reminiscence activities. In the following example the facilitator gave as much time as needed to help Jessica find what she wanted to say. By just affirming that she was still listening, the participant was encouraged to keep going – to try to find the right words. The interaction also identifies how frustrating it can be for people with dementia to join in and contribute when words are difficult to find.

Facilitator: Mmm.

Jessica: I want to do it, but I am slow. And that is the main problem I think, that I am slow at doing these things. I know how to do it, but it doesn't come.

Facilitator: Mmm hmm.

Jessica: I am slow to get that done, and I keep thinking about it, but it is not coming as quickly as I wanted to, and I am slowly exasperated.

Facilitator: Mmm.

The facilitator also needs to be aware of his/her own spirituality, to be comfortable with the types of questions asked in spiritual reminiscence. Questions such as:

- What gives you most meaning in your life?
- What does spirituality mean for you?
- What makes you feel happy or sad?
- What has brought you joy?
- What do you look forward to as you come near the end of your life?

Questions of God and religion were also asked in the groups, and facilitators had to be comfortable with their own spirituality so they could facilitate these topics in discussion (see chapter 15). One facilitator in the study decided not to continue facilitating a group as, although she felt this was important work and she attended church regularly, she did not feel comfortable speaking about religion with others.

An essential beginning for group work is respect by the group facilitator for the group members and a willingness to meet them where they are in their life journeys. The skills used in small groups are those used by the helping professions – first, active listening and being really present with the participants. Effective facilitation of group participation includes using appropriate and open-ended questions and then allowing space and silence while the individual reflects. It includes the use of paraphrasing, unconditional acceptance and the skills of focusing and summarising.

In spiritual reminiscence, it is best to focus on the meaning of events and experiences in the lives of the participants rather than simply on the description of the events remembered. This moves the conversation to a deeper level and enables a review of life meaning. Spiritual reminiscence is one of the spiritual tasks of ageing, and as such an important component of the life journey; it is so much more than simply an activity.

Value for participants and staff

The results from the statistical analysis identified that there were some behaviour changes over the weeks of the groups, especially those lasting 24 weeks. But we were looking for more than that. What did participants get from the groups? Was this an activity that needed to be incorporated into the fabric of the aged care facility? Did participants enjoy the discussions and want to keep the groups going? Could using spiritual reminiscence help to bring about a culture change in the facility that resulted in increased respect for people with dementia?

The following excerpt comes from one of the 24-week groups. During the period of this group one of the participants, John, had died. His wife was also in the group and continued to participate after his death. She often talked about the support she received from the group.

Facilitator: I think we might be finished.

Bronwyn: We might be.

Facilitator: And this is the last time we're meeting – for the purpose of recording, do you want to put on the tape, do you want to say anything about this group and what this group had meant to you?

Margaret: It's meant a lot to me, I've enjoyed it – if you can speak about what you like and what you don't like – no, I think it's very good, I'd like to see more of it.

Bronwyn: I have enjoyed it, immensely, especially when John was here – he used to like to talk.

Margaret: Yes.

Bronwyn: I don't know whether he was always right in what he said but I enjoyed listening to everybody.

In another of the 24-week groups, participants spoke of the pleasure they had from the group and how it helped them to develop relationships. The facilitator makes the comment that she was surprised at how participants responded to the questions – and she had known each of the participants for some time in the aged care facility.

Facilitator: Well we'll start today, um, I'm going to ask you if you want to comment, err, make some comment on what the group has meant to you, coming here and gathering together?

Claire: I think it's tops. Lovely.

Daphne: I think it's all drawn us closer together and we're all beginning to understand our different ways in life, and err helps us to talk about it. Whereas probably in times past we haven't been able to be able to express these things, but I think it helps us all.

Facilitator: What a beautiful thing to say, Daphne. That's always amazing to me how these questions I'm asking would make some young people run a mile, and you've been able to give lots of answers that have been very precious. What do you think about the group, Claire?

Claire: Well, it's helped me to think about things and especially about things I haven't thought about for a while, you know things come up that we remind or something.

Facilitator: That's lovely. Anyone else have a say, to how they feel being part of this group?

Don: It certainly helped me in the realisation that there are other people who held very similar feelings and who when they have a friendly hand stretched out to them, who are not afraid to express that, and therefore make it quite clear to all in the group that it's not one person alone, but all of us together who feel like that. And we look forward to the continuance of those good feelings, even if we don't have the opportunity of meeting and discussing as we are doing now.

The reminiscence groups helped to support participants in a way that was not often experienced in the facilities. Even staff who had known participants for a number of years were surprised at how people with dementia could communicate and participate in the groups. Once given the time, opportunity and support, those with dementia could discuss quite complex concepts and derive pleasure from the interactions.

Summary

Sound communication techniques are essential in the care of older people with dementia. People with dementia are dependent on those around them to reinforce and enhance their sense of self and identity. If there is no response from our conversations then very soon all conversation will cease. In this chapter we have discussed the use of spiritual reminiscence groups as a way to enhance communication between staff and residents and among residents. The spiritual reminiscence groups were most effective when the facilitator was flexible, listened carefully and was skilled at drawing out responses from participants. The use of elderspeak and patronising conversations demonstrates lack of respect and can lead to loss of identity for older people with dementia. Communication is often reduced because there is the commonly held view that those with dementia cannot contribute to a meaningful conversation. By taking positive steps to enhance communication through spiritual reminiscence, we can tap into the core of the person and help to make their life more meaningful.

13

Making Connections

Admission to an aged care facility generally means that the older person has to leave all that is familiar. This includes their home, pets and private space, but also includes leaving behind friends. In this older population, moving away from a neighbourhood can mean dislocation from friends – especially as people may not be able to drive or use public transport. When we visited an aged care facility, we frequently noticed that, while there were many activities within the facilities to engage people, all too frequently people were seated around the room, often with TV or radio at full volume. These surroundings reduce the capacity for people to engage with other residents. Goffman (1961) contended that just being in an institution causes a number of changes and challenges to people, leading to a loss of self. These included being treated all the same, having restricted access to the outside and loss of possessions, roles and autonomy. Kitwood (1997) refers to Meacher (1972), who suggested that the institution of residential care was enough to 'drive people demented'. Kitwood identified specific behaviours that reinforced the patriarchal and sometimes unintentionally callous care when describing his 'malignant social psychology'. So, how do people with dementia make new friends and develop new relationships in aged care? This chapter considers how older people in residential care develop new relationships, maintain long-term relationships and respond to the group work from the spiritual reminiscence groups.

Challenges of connecting with people who have dementia

Part of being human is having relationships. As we have said in previous chapters, the sense of identity is closely related to interaction with others. Kitwood wrote that personhood, or that sense of self, is only provided within the context of mutually recognised, respecting and trusting relationships (Kitwood and Bredin 1992). At one level, as the cognitive function of the person with dementia declines, their personhood can only be upheld and affirmed by others, such as family and carers. And yet, at another level, it seems that perhaps we may be too ready to become 'paternalistic' and 'do for' the person with dementia while they still have considerable reserves of capacity to connect verbally with others. It is a delicate balance which requires a continual testing and affirming with the person: 'What can you do and say?' 'What is hard for you?' 'How can we help best?' One of the most difficult routes to take is for well-meaning care providers to simply observe and best guess what the person can or can't do, without asking and checking with the person. Also, it takes longer for a person with cognitive difficulties to respond to questions, sometimes 5–6 seconds (see chapter 12), and this compounds the difficulties of trying to find out what the person can do. It is important to realise that the person may well be able to indicate their wants and needs, when given sufficient time and support. Many assumptions are made as to what people with dementia can't do; we have found it far more productive to work from the view of what people with dementia can do – and say.

Our analysis of many hours of both individual in-depth interviews and small group sessions of spiritual reminiscence provide direct evidence of the ways in which people with dementia speak and interact with others. Their ability to connect with others can be surprising, and given a supported environment, where they feel un-pressured to speak, they may often enter into meaningful conversation, even when they have low cognitive capacity. At the same time, we have noticed that, where factual information is required of them, their ability to respond declines. One of the facilitators made an interesting comment during the final week of a 24-week group: 'That's always amazing to me how these questions I'm asking would make some young people run a mile, and you've been able to give lots of answers that have been very precious.' Although she had worked in the facility and known the participants for a number of years, she was still taken aback by how participants responded to the group work. We would like to think that in future her interactions with all people with dementia would now be enhanced by her experience.

This raises an important point about relationship that applies to people who have dementia and to others who experience communication difficulties, for instance those with Down's syndrome or those who have strokes and experience dysphasia. As we have discussed in previous chapters, there is frequently an assumption that people with dementia cannot respond to conversations that engage in meaning or emotion, or that are of a spiritual nature. It can readily be seen in the examples that we provide of relationship and connecting that, given patience and understanding rather than being condescending, these people can connect with others and develop new relationships.

Meaning and relationship among people who have dementia

During in-depth interviews, when we asked people with dementia where they found meaning, it was most often through relationship. This of course is very much as it is for any human being. Relationship and connection with other people is vitally important for humans. Studies into attachment demonstrated the importance of closeness and relationship for humans (Bowlby 1973). The main difference for those with dementia is in those with more advanced dementia, as it becomes more difficult to remember names and exact relationships with significant people in their lives. Sometimes they will confuse an adult child for a parent, or talk to an adult child about their own child whom they love, but seem not to realise that they are speaking to that very person. This can be hard for the adult child, who may feel unrecognised, perhaps even discounted, and may wonder what benefit there is in continuing to visit. And yet, it is through relationship that people with dementia are able to connect with others and find meaning in their very existence. Hughes, Louw and Sabat (2006, p.35) note that 'people with dementia have to be understood in terms of relationships, not because this is all that is left to them, but because this is characteristic of all our lives'.

The importance of relationship for people with dementia became real to Elizabeth through, first, her continuing journey with Christine Bryden (Boden), from the time of her diagnosis of dementia, and second, from her journey with her own mother, even though this journey was from a distance of more than 700 kilometres.

When my mother, who had dementia, was still alive, and I would tell people that I was going to visit her, in the nursing home in another state, about eight hours' drive away, I would often be asked: 'Does she recognise you?' To me that was a hard question; in fact, it was the wrong question. The expected answer and indeed the unspoken answer was that if she did not recognise me, then there was no point in visiting.

The terrible context of this question and answer was the focus of it. It begged my purpose in visiting. Was my visit in order to test my mother, to see if she 'still recognised' me?

Rather, it was important to set my visit in another context altogether; my visit was to spend time with my mother. I knew she was vulnerable, and I did not expect her to be able to sit up and say: 'Hello, Elizabeth, and how are you today?'

Often our visit consisted of eye contact and touch, and I would speak of things that I knew were of interest to her. I admit it was not easy, but it was important to me still to continue to visit.

As with people who are cognitively competent, people with dementia have a range of family experiences; Anita spoke of the preciousness of her adopted son.

Interviewer: Your family is important.

Anita: Indeed.

Interviewer: Yeah.

Anita: At the moment.

Interviewer: Yes, yes.

Anita: Very much.

Interviewer: Who, who have you got of your own family at the moment?

Anita: Er, a wonderful son.

Interviewer: Yes.

Anita: We adopted him.

Interviewer: Mmm.

Anita: My husband allowed me to adopt him and er (*pause*) he didn't say anything except that he would like to see me with a young one and then he muttered something about I suppose you won't have anything for (*laughs, missed words*) or kin, just briefly, more or less to himself, which is understandable because he was a very well educated and very everything, he was quite a special man that, but he grew to be very proud of this boy.

Interviewer: Mmm.

Anita: And er (*pause*) and he [her husband] said once, he was in hospital when he was wearing out, was full of men in, in the (*missed word*) room, and we were going and er (*pause*) I, you know, I went out first and he was following me and er I heard him say, at the top of his voice because he didn't hear very well at that stage, good-looking fellow my son.

Some also mentioned long-lasting friendships and, in particular, friends made while doing nursing training. When these women first became nurses their training included living in residences provided by their training hospitals, and close bonds formed there seemed to last a lifetime.

On the other hand, Regina admitted to having no close friends when asked about friends and family:

> **Regina:** I have not got a big family there, so that is awkward, and I have not got, I've got friends, but they are not close to me, and they are further apart and I am here and, yes, but I am quite happy to be here and I love to go walking and I have not got a great deal to do, and I like reading.

June seemed able to speak in the general content area of the questions, but not to give real answers to the questions, even in a broad area of inquiry. The question was not about family or friends, but more broadly about where she received emotional and spiritual support. At one level, it is quite possible that she was really answering the question, as she may have been referring to the staff of the facility where she lived, who provided such support for her:

> **Interviewer:** Um, I wonder if you would like to tell me about the emotional and spiritual supports that you have in your life now. What kinds of supports do you have?
>
> **June:** Well I have it all around this area here, and here, and apart from that I don't really remember any of them. I was a long way out.
>
> **Interviewer:** So who would be the most important people in your life that give you support and...
>
> **June:** Well I think we went through it with everybody, you know, well we sort of worked with one another and...

She went on to speak more of family in the questions that addressed relationships. June's visual problems also restricted her movements. Thus her isolation was compounded by the two aspects of dementia and vision loss.

> **Interviewer:** Ah, so the most important people, relationships in your life.
>
> **June:** Yeah I think so.
>
> **Interviewer:** Yes.
>
> **June:** Most people I've owned.
>
> **Interviewer:** Yes, ah ha. Right, and what about family and friends now?
>
> **June:** Oh I'm just on my own on the moment, because err I'm the last one home, I go home, they see me when they see me; I see them when

I see them, you know. So it's not very often, it just depends on how we can get together, that sort of thing.

In the very first weekly meeting of one of the groups, Don, when asked where he found meaning, said:

Don: The affection, the affection and love of my close relatives, like my son and my granddaughter who have spent such a long time looking after me, while I have been here, and whose companionship has brightened me up when I have been feeling very depressed.

Don had a diagnosis of dementia but an MMSE score of 29. In many ways he was still able to articulate his needs readily but he was still unable to live on his own. His family was obviously important to him. On the other hand, not all of the participants in this same group felt the need for spending time with others.

Daphne: I am not a visitor, I am a loner.

Facilitator: You are a loner.

Daphne: They have all invited me, but I, somebody says come and have a cup of coffee with me, my answer is always no thank you.

Facilitator: Oh.

Claire: It's hard to catch you I think in the lounge.

Facilitator: Do you go to the lounge very often?

Claire: No dear.

Daphne: No, nor do I.

Facilitator: Do you like your room best?

Claire: I am happy there.

The following excerpt from the same session (week two) illustrates both the satisfaction of being alone, and at the same time the participants' awareness of their memory loss. These people spoke quite spontaneously about memory loss, even explaining this to the group facilitator. Note that Daphne has a high MMSE score (30) but also has a diagnosis of dementia.

Facilitator: And, Claire, do you like being by yourself?

Claire: Oh yes, I am not hard to please in that way. I am quite happy.

Facilitator: And, Claire, what about when you have a visitor in your room? I think you had a visitor this morning.

Claire: Can't remember.

Daphne: A lot of us have got short-term memory, we can tell you what happened 60 years ago.

Claire: I have got the most dreadful short-term memory, short term. It's most embarrassing sometimes. (*laughs*)

Facilitator: I was speaking to your daughter this morning. She came to you, J [daughter]. Is that a special time when she comes?

Claire: Oh yes. Yes.

During week two of the spiritual reminiscence groups the research assistant recorded the following observations and comments made by the research assistant during the group session:

> Claire has only one daughter, who visits her. Hetty points to Claire and says: 'she's such a nice person', referring to the daughter. When she realised what she had said could have been ambiguous, she added, pointing again to Claire, 'and so is she'. All participants laugh at this.
>
> They are all attentive to each other and enjoying the conversation. Three group members agree they like their own company and don't mind being alone.
>
> After the group ended, the facilitator said that she was most surprised by Claire. Normally she would not attend social functions or activities, even when encouraged to by staff, but stayed in her room. If she watched TV in the common room she did not engage with others. Now in the group she is sharing and animated in her discussions, and obviously enjoying the conversation and company of the others. The facilitator was amazed at the marked difference.

Although the group had been going only two weeks, participants were interacting, developing relationships and enjoying the sessions.

Hetty: I have got the best daughter I could want.

Facilitator: Oh beautiful. That must be a beautiful relationship, very close, daughter and mother.

Hetty: Oh yes, I don't know, lost my train of thought really.

Facilitator: Oh lovely. So anybody else want to speak about chatting to people? How you like to chat if you have a visitor or if you go out.

Don: You have got to have a common interest, otherwise you can't really chat about anything.

Louise: Well I have lots of, they come, the boys come, and you know, it just goes on and on.

Facilitator: I think you have got a grandchild called Brad, haven't you?

Louise: Yes. But they are all to me, yes.

Facilitator: Tell us something about him, tell us about Brad.

Louise: Brad.

Facilitator: Your Brad.

Louise: Oh I don't know whether I could now, really.

Facilitator: Never mind. Do you know how old he is now?

Louise: Pardon?

Facilitator: Do you know how old he is?

Louise: Oh you have got me now.

Facilitator: That's okay, I don't know myself.

Louise: No, no. Oh I can't talk now.

Facilitator: That's alright, that's lovely. So your sons come to visit you.

It is clear in this last excerpt that Louise was unable to gather facts together, but she was able to respond to more general questions. Early in the conversation she was able to join in by agreeing that 'the boys come' when asked about visitors; however, she seemed to excuse herself from the continuing conversation, as she replied, 'Oh I can't talk now.' It was the concrete concepts that she could not articulate.

The importance of relationship was emphasised in the following excerpt:

Facilitator: Mmm. Speaking of visiting, I'm just remembering, Rose, you have got some special visitors today, haven't you, this evening?

Rose: My daughter.

Facilitator: Do you want to tell us about that?

Rose: Well she's the only one that I've got. I think a lot of her. Comes to see me every night when she can but the children, grandchildren got something on that she has got to go to, but she's coming tonight, and I miss her if she doesn't come. She's very close to me.

There is sadness in the following material from the same session on relationship. The facilitator supports Rose in the conversation. Rose has trouble remembering her sister's address, and maybe some of the details, but the sense of wanting to connect is strong, and illustrates the importance of relationship, or connecting, for these people with dementia:

Facilitator: Beautiful. And Rose?

Rose: I have only got one sister alive, and my husband and all his family died, and I am the only one living out of that family. I have got a sister, sister-in-law, she is only, well she is, she has got TB, just got TB, been in hospital and had the operate, says she is going to be alright, but I feel sorry for her because the woman, her husband's gone. She is all alone.

Facilitator: Where is she living, Rose?

Rose: She lives in Surrey somewhere, I think I have the address but I have forgotten it. Yes, she's a nice girl. She worked for a long time. She married a doctor. She got divorced and she married this doctor, and he died about seven years ago, so she's on her own. But she has got a son of her own, and she has got two, two grandchildren. But she don't make friends very easily, she is a funny girl in some ways.

Facilitator: Do you feel you would like to support her a little bit?

Rose: Hmm. She can't come and see me and I can't go and see her. (*getting upset*)

Facilitator: It's a long way away, Rose, isn't it?

Rose: Yes. I feel she is lonely...

The frustration of actually managing to make contact with family was the focus of this excerpt from Beverley's interview. This raises practical problems of how Beverley can be helped to make contact with her family. Would it be feasible? How might staff assist? Perhaps this is a point where pastoral care providers or recreational activity officers could assist.

Beverley: My family are fairly, family, I have a sister who I most, lives in Australia, we came from Ceylon, and Barbara, my sister, she married a man who took her to, to America, she is in Boston now.

Interviewer: Hmm.

Beverley: So she has been there the same time as we have been here. And we were very close sisters, and I miss her. Now especially, it something that I am missing her, things that we do together. And I am slow to put things together. Why haven't I thought about this all this time, why am I thinking so much about her now? And her husband is already in a hospital for some time, and she was worried about that, and I had been putting off, I wrote her a long letter, and got a reply for that, but that was weeks ago, and I have not had a, I should be writing back to her, or phoning or something to ask her how her husband is, but I am slow then.

Interviewer: Mmm.

Beverley: I want to do it, but I am slow. And that is the main problem I think, that I am slow at doing these things. I know how to do it, but it doesn't come.

Interviewer: Mmm hmm.

Beverley: I am slow to get that done, and I keep thinking about it, but it is not coming as quickly as I wanted to, and I am slowly exasperated.

Interviewer: Mmm.

The importance of relationship, but also not feeling that she had anyone she could share deeply with, was an issue for Martha (in-depth interview only). The fact that she had a 'fantastic' son and daughter did not mean that she could share with them.

Interviewer: Oh, uh okay, who do you share things with, who can you talk to?

Martha: Well, I don't talk personally, talk personally to anybody, except my bank, but I have got nothing there to upset me, or, talk about very much. You know, we are just past all that, got no worries, or anything, so.

Interviewer: It's a good time of life?

Martha: It is a good time of life. Except that I am getting old, and I know there is not much longer, but I don't think about it. I don't dwell on it. No, I am quite happy, and I have got a fantastic son and a daughter and they are very good to me, and I suppose I have been good to them in my time too, so I am very happy. That's the main thing. But I keep very good health, that is the main thing.

Una found it hard not to be near her family, and she said she had no fears but missed her family 'very much'.

Interviewer: Do you have any fears? Do you have any fears in your life?

Una: No I don't think so dear, I've people have been very kind to me and very good and my... Yeah I'm missing my family very much.

Interviewer: What are the hardest things in your life now?

Una: Um, I suppose not having my family around me. Hmm. Hmm. They do come in occasionally. I've only been here what six weeks or something, not very long. Uh hmm.

Forgiveness

Not many mentioned anything about forgiveness, but Mary seemed to be expressing that something had not been able to be resolved prior to the death of one or more of her relatives. The need for closure through confession, forgiveness and reconciliation may be important unfinished business, even for people who have dementia. This process may be used in spiritual reminiscence, but may be more helpful on a one-on-one basis, rather than within a group setting, as usually these issues are very personal. Analysis of the rest of Mary's in-depth interview indicated that she had let go of any resentments or hurt from the past. The following excerpt is from the in-depth interview:

Interviewer: Now, are there any things that you worry about?

Mary: Worry about?

Interviewer: Yes.

Mary: Oh I don't know, I don't know of them. There's not. No. Oh see, most of my family are dying off now, but they're old.

Interviewer: Yep, and you're still here.

Mary: Hmm?

Interviewer: And you're still here?

Mary: Oh well that's right and I don't know why.

Interviewer: Do you worry about that sometimes?

Mary: No, but I would like, there are some things I can't, what will I say, fix up, because from ones I want to in the family speak to are gone.

Interviewer: Yeah. Yes.

Mary: See I'm really on my own and it's not so good.

Interviewer: Hmm, yeah, yeah.

Mary: Now I had an uncle die down the (*missing words*) he was 90 something, but oh, um, I don't think it's bad to live that long.

Interviewer: Yeah. Yes, I think I hear what you're saying. Yep, that there are some downsides to living longer.

Mary: Oh yes.

Loss of relationships

Loss of relationship for elderly people in residential care, whether they have dementia or not, can occur from separation from loved ones through physical separation, perhaps not having access to transport or living at a distance, or, as so often happens, through loss of the loved one through death. In the following example, from an in-depth interview, the resident, Maureen, is 95 years of age and her adult child is unable to drive to visit. Public transport deficiencies may also prevent visits. A generation ago this age would have been unusual, but not now.

> **Interviewer:** Now the first thing I would like to ask you is what is it that means, what means most to you in your life now?
>
> **Maureen:** Well, lying here an answer, because I have no one on the south side, I have two daughters, and my eldest daughter and husband has heart trouble and he can't drive, and she can't get here because she can't drive.
>
> **Interviewer:** How old is she?
>
> **Maureen:** 75.
>
> **Interviewer:** And you are?
>
> **Maureen:** 95.
>
> **Interviewer:** That's a great age.

It is often thought that people with dementia do not know when someone has died, and as they cannot remember, then the loss of relationship is not comprehended. Some people with dementia will ask over and over again for a loved one who has died. Sometimes they will go back to their childhood days and talk as if they are still children and their parents are alive. We wonder if this is more to do with seeking for reminders of connections with loved ones that we have found to be so important for these people. Both the individual in-depth interviews and group sessions were valuable sources of information on grief among the participants in the study. The following excerpt is from an in-depth interview; note that Janet lost her train of thought part way through the answer and asked what she was saying. Gently reminded by the interviewer, she continued with her response:

> **Interviewer:** Now what about grief? Have you...
>
> **Janet:** Grief?
>
> **Interviewer:** Grief, yes have you experienced much in the way of grief?
>
> **Janet:** I think everybody at some time or the other has had a little bit of grief, say they have been going to work, and then work (*pause*) for instance, I know, some people don't know. (*pause*) Ah. (*pause*) What was I saying?
>
> **Interviewer:** About grief.

Janet: Oh, grief. Some people have grief when there is not really grief. If it is grief for those sort of people it is for themselves, it is not for everybody, and there is a difference, see?

Interviewer: So have you experienced, what have been the biggest situations of grief that you have experienced?

Janet: Death in the family, I felt grief, mostly. You have enough of your own, without broadcasting it, know what I mean, and then sometimes you have it, and you should not have it, it is none of your business, but you can't help that there is grief.

The following excerpt identifies how, even many years after the loss of a relationship through death, the memories are still very real and continue to evoke sadness. Bronwyn lost her sister when she was a young adult, yet when asked about sadness in her life this was still the most important.

Bronwyn: Oh I remember with sadness the death of my sister who was just a few years older than me.

Interviewer: Um.

Bronwyn: It was a great loss to me, because we were very close, and it's something that has always been with me and err she was only the really young one, and err I don't mean to be sad but it has been a great sadness, we continue on with life, but that's it.

Interviewer: It is remembering with sadness isn't it? Hmm, that's what you're doing. And how old was she?

Bronwyn: She was 23.

Interviewer: 23, hmm. Were you married at that stage Bronwyn?

Bronwyn: No.

Interviewer: Thank you for sharing that. It's hard to remember with sadness and share it, but that's what we're asking.

Loneliness

There were a number of occasions when participants talked about when they felt lonely. Loneliness was discussed as part of the spiritual reminiscence group. Amy was obviously very outgoing and managed to find the comfort of friends in the aged care facility. She is also very philosophical about being lonely and admits that it is 'something you have to learn to live with'.

Amy: No, I think that is one of the advantages of a place like this, where as if you were at home, like stay at home, if you are, then I think the loneliness could be quite acute, whereas here, well if you walk just up and down the corridor for a while, you will meet up with someone you could talk to, or have a joke with, or something.

Facilitator: So are you saying it is really up to you?

Amy: Well it is never completely up to one person I suppose, you've got to get that.

Facilitator: Two way.

Amy: Yes, but…well I think personal loneliness in your life is something you have to learn to live with, and we all seem to have to face a certain amount of it, don't we?

Anita, on the other hand, seems to find it more difficult to establish relationships in the aged care facility. She admits that it is her fault. Amy adds to the conversation again with her philosophical approach 'acceptance is the thing'.

Facilitator: How would you feel about that, Anita? Do you feel lonely here? Do you ever feel lonely?

Anita: I think so, but I don't notice, I don't think that anyone goes to me, it's probably my fault though.

Facilitator: So even though there are people here and you go and join them at lunchtime and teatime, and pass the time of day with them at the table, you don't really spend other times with them.

Anita: No.

Facilitator: Right, so you do have periods of loneliness here.

Anita: Oh well, I don't know if you can do anything about that. That's, it's being human I suppose.

Amy: Acceptance is the thing, isn't it?

In the following example, Karen described the sadness she felt at having no one. Although she was in an aged care facility with company around her all the time, she still felt as if she had no one. This can be quite a common feeling – it is difficult to establish new relationships, and for some older people, especially those with dementia, it is too difficult. Violet is supportive – within the spiritual reminiscence groups participants helped to be there for each other.

Facilitator: What about you, Karen, what do you look back on with sadness? When you look back at your life, what do you remember with sadness? What makes you sad?

Karen: That I have nobody. Nobody.

Violet: That can be sad too.

In the following interaction about friends and loneliness, Ben and Amy regret the loss of the ability to read. It becomes more important for them to be able to connect in other ways as they can no longer get the pleasure or connection they used to through reading.

Anita: There are friends in books.

Facilitator: That's right, very true...

Ben: And you can lose yourself entirely, that's what happened to me.

Facilitator: Because you love reading, don't you, especially if it is a book that really gets your attention.

Ben: I used to love reading, but I, it's gone...

Facilitator: You can't concentrate on it, Ben?

Ben: Yes, to a certain degree.

Facilitator: I guess you miss that.

Ben: Yes.

Amy: I'm the same, I always loved reading most of my life, then suddenly I lost interest in it.

Anita: What was that?

Facilitator: Reading, Amy lost interest in reading.

Group support and connections

There was great advantage working in groups for the spiritual reminiscence project. All participants were interviewed individually before entering the project – and it was very interesting to see how they developed during the six- or 24-week group sessions. Participants shared many of their problems, especially around memory loss, and they had the chance to think about other things that had formed part of their lives. Listening to people with dementia means listening not to just the happy times, but being prepared to deal with anger, anxiety, fear and sorrow. Within the groups each participant was very supportive and they all helped each other. Participants in many of the groups, especially those lasting 24 weeks, developed good friendships. The following interaction occurred in week ten of the sessions. A number of participants join in with the conversation in response to the question 'What is it like growing older?' There is much interaction and contribution to the conversation from all the participants. There are aspects of humour and acceptance of getting older. There is also acceptance of death – with participants saying they do not want to reach 100.

Facilitator: Okay, what's it like growing older?

Rose: Ooh, what's it like growing older?

Facilitator: Yes.

Rose: Oh.

Hetty: Well you have got to make the best of it.

Daphne: Mmm.

Hetty: Forget about getting older.

Daphne: Forget about it.

Rose: You can't do things you want to do when you get older, like go dancing.

Claire: I'm loving it.

Facilitator: Loving it, well, party girl talking.

Hetty: I never thought I'd get to 90.

Facilitator: That's not very old is it?

Daphne: You are 90?

Hetty: Yes.

Daphne: Yes.

Hetty: And I never thought I would get there.

Daphne: Mmm.

Hetty: My family, the young ones, reckon I will get to 100.

Facilitator: Get to 100?

Hetty: Yes.

Facilitator: Yes, I reckon you will.

Rose: I don't want to live to 100.

Hetty: No, I don't particularly.

Rose: You have to go the way you want to get out.

The following excerpt is from the same group. Again it is interesting to note how participants care and support each other in this interaction. Participants, despite their dementia, remembered the number of weeks that Hetty had been absent from lunch and were concerned about how she was progressing. Hetty had started to return to the dining room for her meals – this was obviously a good milestone that had been noted. This interaction took place after 15 weeks of the group meeting.

Facilitator: You right? You look very tired, Hetty.

Daphne: Yes.

Facilitator: Would you like me to take you back now?

Hetty: Oh no.

Facilitator: You'll be right?

Claire: Hetty hopes she is going to be okay.

Daphne: Yes, I know there is a lot of them like that.

Claire: She has got that rattly chest.

Daphne: Yes, I know she has.

Facilitator: You are doing well, Hetty.

Claire: Each day getting better.

Hetty: Yes.

Daphne: Started to come to the dining table again, which is nice to see, because so many are away.

Facilitator: Oh that's great, Hetty, I did not know that.

Daphne: Yes I had not seen her for weeks, a couple of weeks.

Hetty: Sometimes I, I don't feel as good as I could.

Daphne: Some people can get about better than others. I can just manage. A lot of people can't get around very well.

Hetty: I think it is nice how everybody fits here, fits in place.

The following excerpt shows how participants interacted with little assistance from the facilitator during quite a complicated interchange about life when they were younger.

Brenda: What is it like now? What is it like now, with normal sort of people?

Ross: Like normal. The place is gone, people all realise after the war it was just ridiculous to fight each other about religion, and that was the reason, and that is what he thought, and then the Protestants and the Catholics, they all mixed together, and...

Brenda: They made a happy country in a way.

Ross: Yes, and the royal family, they were...and they were head of whatever the church was, this was, so they were always special occasions.

Brenda: Because our royal family go over quite often, don't they, from England.

Ross: Yes.

Brenda: They do.

Ross: And they do the same as the English family, there is no difference.

Facilitator: So things have improved.

Brenda: What, darling?

Facilitator: Things have improved.

Brenda: Oh right, enormously, yes. I am sure they have, don't you? Things have improved. It is not so...hated. That's one thing of a word.

Ross: I remember when I was a little boy, people say what school are you going to, what Catholics, oh yes, Catholics. Nowadays, they would not ask the question. They know it was always the boy at that age is going to school, so why asking the question? Also what is the Catholic supposed to do?

Brenda: Well, it was the last war, of course, that made them all think, wasn't it, really?

Ross: Uh, I think it might have been, yes.

Brenda: Yes, yes.

Ross: And it was, and the last war, um, the, did a lot of good work, because they were not recognised by any, they were just dressed in normal clothes, not in their uniform, the ones we used to have, right before the war we used to have people dressed up like Nazis from the war, but then war came back and got rid of it.

Brenda: They got rid of the Nazi uniform.

Ross: All of them they did, and they came back to earth again. After the war, it was just, anybody was walking whether it was a Jew, or a

Protestant, you would be grateful for on the street, and this fellow was a Jew, and there were Catholics, that didn't matter.

Brenda: They were normal people, yes.

Ross: We all were.

Summary

Having relationships is part of being human. Establishing relationships or maintaining old ones is particularly difficult in the environment of residential aged care. Often these people are particularly vulnerable when admitted to an aged care facility, having lost life partners, home and friends. Yet those with dementia are able to develop these relationships and grow new ones, if given support and encouragement. The small groups in the spiritual reminiscence programme provided this support and encouragement, demonstrating the importance of relationships to the participants. Some of the participants were confused about the exact nature of relationship with the people they spoke of; however, there was a sense of the importance of these relationships, especially seen in the fondness with which some spoke of their mothers or fathers. 'Knowing' is not simply putting a label of a name onto a person; rather, knowing is a deeper concept. Reports from staff and the research assistants both identify the ways that participants helped each other, both verbally and non-verbally, to interact in a meaningful way.

14

Ritual, Symbol and Liturgy

The spiritual dimension is mediated through relationship, through creation and environment, through the arts and through religion (MacKinlay 2006). This chapter contains material on connections to the spiritual and responses to meaning seen in the participants of the study. This study was not about actual liturgy or the use of rituals or symbols, but about spiritual reminiscence; therefore the study participants spoke about what they engaged in, their memories of church and worship, their current practices of religion and ways of connecting with the spiritual dimension. However, later in the chapter, we do explore the use of ritual and liturgy and continuing spiritual growth in later life, with some strategies that might be incorporated into the spiritual reminiscence process.

To place this chapter in context, it is part of the model of the spiritual tasks and process of ageing (MacKinlay 2001a). The person responds to their life-meaning in ways that support that meaning and in turn affirm meaning for them. Humans are meaning makers by nature, and the use of symbols and rituals can importantly carry and affirm these meanings.

Communities often have corporate symbols and rituals, and, in a secular sense, even a graduation ceremony with all its symbolism can help affirm and support graduates and their families. Community celebrations may be seen at different seasons of the year, when particular rituals will be played out. Religious rituals and symbols are often played out in the context of a liturgy or religious service. These support and affirm meaning, not just of the individual, but to the body of believers. People with dementia need symbols and rituals as much as any other people. Sacks (1985) has written of the story of 'Jimmy' (referred to in detail in chapter 1), a man that Sacks thought had no cognitive abilities, but who could be seen in the chapel coming alive during a service of worship.

Discussion with a chaplain in aged care recently revealed that, in a particular aged care facility, church services had been discontinued in the dementia-specific unit, and those who were thought to be 'capable of understanding what was going on' would now be taken to a service in another part of the facility.

The chaplain was understandably distressed by this decision, as it is now well known that the emotional and spiritual dimensions remain in ways that allow these people to connect with meaning long after they lose the ability to speak, and it is through these means that some continue to connect with others at times throughout the progress of this disease.

We might hope that general understandings of dementia may have increased in the community, and especially within the aged care sector in recent years, to include the new understandings of the nature of the needs of the person with dementia. These new understandings of the nature of the person who has dementia affirm the benefits of being able to be part of a church service, unless they do not want to attend.

It is important that such services are open and available to people with dementia. People who are thought to be unable to speak may participate in the liturgy, sometimes joining in prayers and singing. They may, like Sacks' Jimmy, come alive during the liturgy. But even if the person does not actively participate, assumptions should not be made about the level of understanding of the person. The person may simply not be able to communicate their level of understanding to those who observe.

Response to meaning may be in many forms, such as through worship, through art, music and poetry or through symbols, drama, prayer and reading of Scripture. Symbols may be religious or secular. There is something about human beings that brings a deep-seated need for connections through symbol and ritual. For those who have no connections with anything of a religious nature, symbols still retain their importance. The importance of symbols lies in their ability to carry meaning for the particular people of a particular culture. Thus the variety of symbols is only restricted by the imagination of the people involved. Effective symbols can be flowers, leaves, pebbles, water, candles, religious symbols, a cross for Christians, prayer mats for Muslims, incense, rosaries and statues for Hindus and Buddhists. Special foods, fasting and ceremonies would fit here too, such as the Muslim observance of Ramadan, and special Jewish festivals (Abdalla and Patel 2010; Barzaghi 2010; Cohen 2010; Rayner and Bilimoria 2010).

This chapter addresses issues of the ways that these people connect with meaning and their God. One example of this relationship with God is seen when the facilitator asked a participant 'So do you feel near to God now, Elma?' and she replied: 'God and I have developed, he is always here.' This comment speaks of a continuing journey, of this person who has dementia, with her God. It speaks of an assurance of God's presence with her.

Of course, not all the people in the study had a relationship with God, and they met their needs for connecting with the spiritual dimension in other ways, as will be seen through the chapter.

Information relating to religious activities was obtained through the group sessions, and no questionnaire was used to elicit data. Thus we have accounts of Bible reading and study, prayer and church attendance, but not the number of times attended. We were attempting to find what worked for these people, rather than keeping a record of frequency of attendance. Thus meaning was deemed to be of more importance than calculating frequency of worship. Memories of early childhood church attendance were still alive for many of these older adults. This cohort of older people had mostly been taken or sent to church and/or Sunday school when they were young. Some of the following were found in the transcripts:

- discussion of the place of ritual and symbols with people who have dementia
- symbols and ritual with older people
- connecting ritual and symbol for people with dementia.

Questions asked during interviews and group sessions focused on the following broad issues:

- Do you have an image of God or some sense of a deity or otherness? *Or, use other words that are meaningful to the group, such as:* What do you think God is like?
- If you hold an image of God, can you tell me about this image?
- Do you feel near to God?
- What are your earliest memories of church, mosque, temple or other worship? Did you attend Sunday school, church or other religious activity when you were young?
- Do you take part in any religious/spiritual activities now – e.g. attend church services, Bible or other religious readings, prayer, meditation?
- How important are these to you?

These questions helped to flesh out the status of the spiritual and religious involvement of the participants. Discussions took place about what they did, memories of early life and church or Sunday school, what it meant to them and, particularly in the small group sessions, they were asked how they prayed, and in what ways this was helpful or not.

The religious and spiritual practices of participants

This first selection from the transcripts is from the initial in-depth interviews. The conversation was mainly about the religious practices of these people. Most of these older adults had a history of church and Sunday school when they were young, even if they had ceased all association with religion in later life. When they were young, the different denominational differences were more pronounced and loyalty to one denomination was usually strong. Unless they had continued to be part of a worshipping community, they would likely have memories of churches where the minister or priest led the worship and there would have been less lay involvement. Some Catholics noted that, when they were young, they always had the Bible read to them, but did not read it themselves, with one woman saying that it was 'filtered' to them through the Sisters. In their youth, there was less overall lay involvement than there is these days, in many denominations. It is with these kinds of backgrounds that we engaged with these participants. Thus there is little that refers to ritual, but much in relation to church services, which could contain rituals, Bible studies and prayer:

> **Interviewer:** Mmm, I'm wondering, now do you, do you read any religious things or do you take part in any Bible studies or, um, meditation or...
>
> **Amy:** Yes, well of course prayer is a form of meditation really, isn't it?
>
> **Interviewer:** Yes.
>
> **Amy:** And er (*pause*) I try to stay as close to God as I possibly can.
>
> **Interviewer:** Yes, that is good.
>
> **Interviewer:** I'd like to take a change in direction now and ask you, do you have a faith then?
>
> **Jane:** I'm Church of England.
>
> **Interviewer:** Yes.
>
> **Jane:** I go to Bible studies.
>
> **Interviewer:** Yes.
>
> **Jane:** I don't go every week. I don't practise faith every week but when I...I go.
>
> **Interviewer:** Now you say you enjoy to go to church and so you go to the services here?

Jane: Yes, they have the services on Sunday. They're there. The services are very nice.

Interviewer: Do you take part in any kind of spiritual or religious kind of activities here now?

Hetty: Yes, I go to church. Yes I enjoyed the church, the ladies that have the service in, quite nice ladies.

Interviewer: Do you take part in any kind of activities here? Do you ever go along to the Communion or church or Bible classes here?

Claire: Uh, no, I don't take any active part in any of those sorts of things, but I go along to services.

Interviewer: Do you ever take part in any kind of spiritual or religious activities here?

Candy: I go to Communion every Friday, I've been this morning, that's all. Oh, sometimes I go to Bible studies. Sometimes, not often.

Rose, in her in-depth interview (below), alluded to a change in her prayer and faith life. It was difficult to pin-point what was happening for her. She seemed hesitant to speak of what she thought God was like, and that she used to have an image of God, but not now, yet she goes to church currently, and she said it has changed for her, but she was not able to say how. To some extent her early church attendance may have been part of what the family did on Sundays, and perhaps she now did not see the need to hold this as part of her life, yet she did still attend church. The interviewer invited a contact with the chaplain, but Rose did not seem to want to follow up on this. During the interview transcript excerpt below, it can be seen that the interviewer gently explored the topic with Rose. This may become a sensitive area, so it is important not to push for religious involvement (although the chaplain would not only be looking at religious matters, but would be concerned about meaning and spirituality in a broad context). Perhaps Rose wanted no more involvement than her weekly attendance, and the change that she experienced would need to remain with her. The fact that she said 'It could come back to me' is worth keeping in mind, in case she later decides that she would like to have a visit from pastoral care. It is important to respect the person's desire for further engagement, or choice for no further engagement. When working with vulnerable people, this is always an important consideration.

Interviewer: Now, I want to take a change of where we are going at the moment, and I want to ask you about whether you have any sense or image of God or some kind of deity or otherness?

Rose: No I haven't. I used to. (*mumbles*)

Interviewer: And what happened?

Rose: I couldn't, I didn't take. (*pause*) I can't speak as well as I used to speak.

Interviewer: Do you go to any of the services here?

Rose: Yes, I go every Friday morning.

Interviewer: And do you enjoy those?

Rose: Yes.

Interviewer: Well that's good.

Rose: I don't feel the same about it.

Interviewer: You don't feel the same about it? Okay, can you tell me a little bit more about how you feel about that now?

Rose: Ooh, to tell you the truth I haven't even thought about that.

Interviewer: You have not really thought about that very much?

Rose: No, not since I have been here, I used to do, I used to go to church, and I was very good. When I was little I used to go to church every Sunday.

Interviewer: That was just part of what you did on Sunday.

Rose: Yes.

Interviewer: So is there a way in which you miss that now?

Rose: Mmm hmm. It's not the same any more.

Interviewer: No, so do you see that you have any spiritual needs?

Rose: Not at the moment.

Interviewer: Not at the moment? Now I am wondering if you have, you say you go to the church services here on a Friday?

Rose: Some weeks, also on the weekend.

Interviewer: Yes, on a Friday.

Interviewer: Do you have any negative memories about anything to do with religion at all?

Rose: Yes I used to go out [on] Sunday, I used to like to go to church, on Christmas and Boxing Day.

...

Rose: I used to be good, I used to go to church and I used to do things with friends, and go to church, I used to enjoy it.

Interviewer: Would you like to be able to do that again? Be able to enjoy church?

Rose: I think it will come back to me.

Interviewer: You think?

Rose: It could come back to me.

Interviewer: Would you like the chaplain to come and visit you?

Rose: I don't know him, do I?

Interviewer: Hmmm?

Rose: I don't know him very well.

Interviewer: Well there is a lady chaplain here at the moment.

Rose: Here? In the church here?

Current spiritual and religious practices were not always what the participants would have hoped for. They shared memories of what they used to do:

Facilitator: Anybody attend any prayer groups, or do prayer as a group?

Claire: Not now, I miss it very much. I used to go every Monday evening, used to be the prayer meeting, and those sort of things, yes I do miss, but I carry them in my memory and in my mind and in my spiritual being and it still means a lot to me 'cause I can remember so much of the past.

Facilitator: Do you take part in any spiritual or religious activity?

Margaret: Well I don't, but I like Bible study, that's about all that I like now. And um I don't think I'm learning a lot about it, but it's interesting. I don't go to church, err I don't know why, I did up till the late years, then I dropped out when things went wrong and um I've never been back to church really to enjoy it. But Bible study I like.

Facilitator: Would you like to say how often you do that?

Margaret: Well, only here once a week, I think it is.

On the other hand, Violet did not wish to attend church, but did so to please her family. She said that she held no belief, and did not take Communion; however, she attended with the family.

Facilitator: So it's your spiritual activity that we're trying to err draw out today. It's not somebody else's.

Violet: As I have said before, I believe in people and how you react to them, and how they react to you. That to me is far more important than any spiritual feeling at all. I go to church with the family as requested, but I would never take Communion because I'm not a hypocrite. That is my...but if the family want to go Christmas Eve, then I'll go with them, or Easter I'll go, not because I believe in it, and I will never take Communion, because that to me is hypocrisy for me, but I don't mind the family doing it. It's not, I mean I do not, but I will not offend the family by refusing to go, that is my attitude to it. But it means nothing to me in myself.

Facilitator: Thank you for that.

Violet: I'm more concerned with my reaction on the people I meet, and their reaction to my responses.

John was another participant who did not appreciate religious activities or beliefs. He appeared happy to be in a group of participants where some of them had a religious faith while others did not. Religious beliefs were discussed openly, and respect was given to the different perspectives of the participants.

Jill, in an in-depth interview, was clear in her opinions about church, and her beliefs were respected.

Interviewer: Right. And you don't go to church or anything now?

Jill: No, that's right. I found a lot of wrongs I didn't agree with. Everybody does that though.

John had a more nuanced view of religion, supporting his wife in attending church, but 'not taking it seriously' himself.

John: Well I've read in a religious area like err atmosphere, and it wasn't until I was 16 or 17 that I shed it all and I forced my way through work and everything else, and then I had six years away. And I saw things during those six years that made me wonder, because one minute you're with your mates and the next minute you're burying them and all that sort of thing. And I've been quite cynical about it ever since, I worry about the family of course, but err religion with me, I go with Joyce to church and appreciate it, but I don't take it seriously. Um, but err I'm not being funny about this but…

Facilitator: Thank you, it's very kind of you to share.

John: I find it hard to, um, because there's things I've seen that I could never reconcile with religion, there's too much and I can see it now. It's one of those lasting impressions of what you've seen and that and err. And err I follow a life which is guided by principles and I appreciate people who are religious and all that sort of thing, but it doesn't affect me. I love my girl and she can be very religious at times, but we go to church together, but err no I can't. I couldn't get up and spruik [speak publically, evangelise or promote] about it or anything like that, because I would say that I am being a damn hypocrite.

Brenda was adamant about her lack of belief in any religious system. Then, surprisingly, she says that she still goes to church, but only for the singing:

Interviewer: And I wonder if I could ask you, do you have a faith or a belief in your life? Do you have a belief system?

Brenda: No. I am very, what can you say, what can you call me? I am very anti all the religious stuff. And I really believe that people overdo it, and if they just get on with their own things, we'd all be far better off.

Interviewer: Right.

Brenda: That's why (*pause*) oh I mean I still go to church.

Interviewer: Oh do you?

Brenda: I still go to church because, in Durham, a church school. So I still go, but only for the singing.

Interviewer: And you really enjoy that?

Brenda: Yes, and I really enjoy that, yes.

Edith does not regard herself as a 'churchgoer' but still likes to attend sometimes. The comment from 'the woman' seemed to classify Edith into a category that she did not want to be placed.

Interviewer: Have you ever, um, have you ever been to church or been involved in any religious things?

Edith: Oh yes, I've been to church, but I am not a churchgoer. Not, I've been since I've been since, I've been down here, the church, they went off one Sunday and asked if I'd like to go, and I said, 'Yes.' And the woman there she said, 'I didn't think you went to church.' I said, 'I don't, but I still believe in it.' I said, 'I still believe in church and that sort of thing.'

I've had one of those church people in here, got to go to church and all that rush. No, I'm not like that, I just keep on going the way I do.

Interviewer: And you keep it with you, do you?

Edith: Yeah, I keep it with me.

Few of these older people seemed to have any idea of meditation, and below is one of the few responses from the small group sessions. Perhaps Bronwyn is saying something about meditation, perhaps not:

Facilitator: Now, um, so you go to church services here. Do you take part in any Bible studies, or Bible readings or...?

Bronwyn: Yes.

Facilitator: Yes?

Bronwyn: Quite a few days I do Bible reading.

Facilitator: And do you do any meditation at all?

Bronwyn: I think a lot.

Facilitator: You think a lot. Yes, within yourself.

Bronwyn: Yes.

Prayer

Prayer forms an important aspect of connecting with God. Prayer may take different forms, and can be related to level of faith, maturity in faith and religious background, including the particular denomination. It can vary in formality and regularity. In earlier studies of cognitively intact older adults (MacKinlay 2001a, 2001b, 2006), a number of participants found their prayer changing as they grew older, and the majority of them prayed. Prayer can be much more than bringing requests and intercessions to God – it can be a listening to God. The changing ways of praying may be an opening to God. Benner (2010) suggests that prayer can become a way of life, rather than just an activity. In the transcripts we looked for evidence of current prayer life, of whether this had changed – and self-awareness of this. We looked to see what importance these people attached to their prayer life and what their prayer meant to them.

PRAYER IN THE IN-DEPTH INTERVIEWS

In this sample of people with dementia, there was a great range of responses to questions of whether they prayed. When asked if she prayed or read the Bible, Claire replied: 'Well I used to, but I'm afraid I don't any more.' Others still prayed; for instance, Candy (MMSE 30) said: 'I pray a lot. Very quietly, very silently.' And also Jane:

Jane: Oh, I pray, I pray every night.

Interviewer: And have you found that over the years that your prayer has changed at all, in any way?

Jane: No, I don't pray as much. When I was younger I'd say prayers and I'd buy a new dress. (*laughing*)

Rose spoke a lot about her spiritual and religious habits; she still attended church and was asked about prayer:

Interviewer: Do you pray?

Rose: Yes.

Interviewer: And would you do that every day, or when you think about it?

Rose: No, I did it in my happy days.

Interviewer: And do you think your prayer life has changed?

Rose: Yes.

Interviewer: In what way?

Rose: I don't think about it any more.

Interviewer: You don't think about it any more?

Rose: No.

Interviewer: So nowadays you might just pray if there was something that you really had a need for. Is that the sort of thing?

Rose: I do, I might just go.

The variations between participants was marked, from those who did not pray at all (most did pray), to some for whom prayer was a way of being. The purpose of prayer varied also, with some using prayer as a way of asking for support, for giving thanks for blessings and good things in their lives, for help for themselves and family members, and also for conversation with God. In an earlier study of independent older people (MacKinlay 2001a), some noted that their prayer had changed over the years, and that now it was becoming more a conversation with God. Sometimes just being with God seemed to be all that was required. Some felt they should be saying the set prayers that they had learnt when they were younger, while others felt comfortable as they were now. Such variations were also present in this study.

The following are three very different responses to the question of prayers. The first, emphatically, Louise (MMSE 4): 'No, I don't.' The second, Carol (MMSE 27): 'I say my prayers, that's it.' The third, Rodney (MMSE 30): 'I am praying all the time: I want help, can hardly breathe, I am asthmatical.' Catherine finds her prayer is much the same over the years. Maureen said: 'Oh yes, I do.' When asked if she found that helpful, she said: 'Oh yes, of course. I have always the Lord to talk to. I don't know if I'm mad or not, but...' Bronwyn acknowledged that prayer formed an important part of her life:

Interviewer: And do you pray often?

Bronwyn: I do, yes. Yes.

Interviewer: About how often would you pray?

Bronwyn: Oh I pray quite a lot, I mean, um, because I feel that I have. I feel that I have things to be so thankful for, and I think sometimes I'm living on borrowed time. But I'm quite prepared for that. It sounds romantic really, but it's not really. That's the way I feel.

In contrast, John (MMSE 25) only prayed when he had a real need to ask for something. Margaret (MMSE 29) and Mary (MMSE 20) were both definite about the importance of prayer, with Mary praying every night, as a long-term habit. George found comfort in prayer. Keryn (MMSE 20) used her rosary beads, while Elvie (MMSE 27) said: 'And if I want to do something I pray about it, it's just as if He's here and then "thy will, Lord, not mine", you know, and there's always it turns out okay.' Doris (MMSE 10), when asked if she prayed, replied: 'No. No.' Helen (MMSE 11) responded by saying: 'I do read the Bible, can't say I pray. I do read the Bible.' It is interesting that she reads the Bible but does not pray, as it is possibly more common to pray than to read the Bible, and if a person does read the Bible, they are likely to pray. So it is difficult to say what is happening there. In the example that follows, it is not possible to be sure of what Maude's habits were in early life, due to her failing memory.

Interviewer: Do you, you've said you go to church, um, do you pray?

Maude: No, not really.

Interviewer: Not really? Have you ever been a pray-er? Have you ever been a person to pray, even your younger days?

Maude: I don't know. I can't remember.

PRAYER IN THE GROUP SESSIONS

Different groups brought forth different amounts of material on prayer. To some extent this could be expected, taking into account the characteristics of the facilitator and the members of a particular group.

In week six of one group the following responses were recorded:

Facilitator: So, about prayer, do you all pray?

Amy: Yes.

Facilitator: Yep.

Amy: Every day.

Facilitator: Yes. Yep.

Ben: Yes.

Facilitator: Do you pray, Ben?

Ben: Not so much that I used to.

Facilitator: Yes, what about you, Anita?

Anita: I keep Him pretty busy.

The following is one of the small group sessions where participants talked about their prayer. Anita expressed her feelings that sometimes God seemed distant; however, she did not stop talking with God.

Facilitator: Hmmm, yes. What about you, Anita, do you, um, do you say a set pray when you pray, or do you just bring whatever is on your mind?

Anita: I just sort of talk.

Amy: Talk to God I call it, talking to God it should be really. When things get really bad I wonder whether he is listening, you know, where are you God?

Facilitator: Yes, that's when you cry out, isn't it?

Anita: I wish there was more opportunities for myself, and in fact I could ask for myself, you know, I visit in my mind. Do you see? Yes I do that.

Within the group sessions, prayer was discussed by the facilitator and group members; the following is one way in which the facilitator fruitfully engaged with all group members:

Facilitator: I am just going to ask you, Louise, one more question, um, Louise, do you remember any of the prayers from your childhood?

Louise: Yes, I do really, we were very, quite kind, you know, and we, that was all what it was. It was always on me, and, really.

Facilitator: Um, has there been a time when you have doubted that God was there?

Louise: No. Never have, to me anyway. Yes.

Facilitator: Louise, I just want to ask one special question.

Louise: Yes.

Facilitator: Um, do you remember, would you remember the Lord's Prayer, Our Father?

Louise: Yes, I could.

Facilitator: Do you remember that prayer, Rose?

Rose: Yes.

Facilitator: Do you remember that prayer, Our Father, Hetty? Do you remember that prayer, Our Father?

Hetty: Yes, yes.

Facilitator: I think Don is nodding.

In the following excerpt, the facilitator explores the possibility of someone praying with the group members. Claire had raised an issue that she was concerned about, and the facilitator wanted to know if it was alright for her to pray with her. The facilitator already knew the group members and how they felt about spiritual matters, so it was an appropriate step to take, but it is noted that she did not just go ahead and pray without ensuring that she had Claire's consent:

Facilitator: Claire, would, how would you feel if someone came to pray with you? Would you like that, is that something that you would like, or you are not used to that?

Claire: Oh no, I'm...I like to pray dear, especially with someone that I know has the same sort of feeling, you know, you can tell, can't you?

Facilitator: Thank you, Claire, that's lovely. Hetty, did you want to say anything about the power of prayer before we finish?

Hetty: Yes. I think about the...and I like to, to pray, and I think it helps, helps me.

In the next group session it can be seen that the group members are interacting more with each other, and the facilitator stays in the background:

Facilitator: Thank you for that memory as well Don. Gentle Jesus. Did anyone else learn that prayer when they were young, Gentle Jesus?

Daphne: Well it's a hymn, I do believe.

Don: It's a fairly well-known prayer isn't it?

Facilitator: Did you learn that prayer, Claire?

Claire: Yes, dear.

Facilitator: Was that the first one you learnt?

Claire: No. Our Father which art in heaven, hallowed be thy name. Thy kingdom come, thy will be done. Give us this day our daily bread.

Daphne: Forgive us. Go on.

Claire: No, you finish it.

Daphne: And forgive us our trespasses as we forgive those who trespass against us. Yeah. We didn't learn it not to be recited off by heart you know. I'm learning it all now from the cook now when we go to chapel, 'cause I don't know it. People can recite everything, but I've got to strain my eyes to find what word is next.

Facilitator: Louise, can I ask you if you know that prayer, Gentle Jesus? Have you learnt that prayer?

A week later, in the same group, the facilitator asked the group members the following question, which elicited the following conversation from Rose who had contributed little to the group on this topic previously. Note the sensitive way that the facilitator encourages Rose to express herself, even when she has difficulty with the words:

Facilitator: Anyone else want to say whether this group's made a difference from the way you feel about God?

Rose: I don't know, but I think I seldom to go but I don't know when. I've gone from one to the other. I used to go to church and all, but I don't know what stopped me, I got ill or something and…

Facilitator: Can you express, Rose, thank you for being so honest, um, can you, would you like to say, ah you've gone from one to the other, where do you want to be, do you know?

Rose: Well I want to go back to where I was.

Facilitator: Which is where?

Rose: Oh I used to be happy, I used to, I used to pray and everything else, but I don't pray now.

Facilitator: Do you mean, are you saying that you would like to start praying again?

Rose: Yes, but I, something has stopped me, I don't know what it is, but it does.

It is noted that Rose was referred to earlier in the chapter as not praying. Following the end of this session the following is recorded from the research assistant journal:

> When the tape turned off, the facilitator offers to pray for Rose. She says 'yes' and appears to be grateful and moved by this, crying more openly.
> The group holds hands and the facilitator leads the group in prayer.
> They stay for a while talking about the freedom they feel in being able to talk with each other and how they feel close to each other in faith.

Church attendance and changes over the years

It is possible to see stages of growth and change in the spiritual dimension across the lifespan (Fowler 1981). Fowler sees most older people at stages 3–5 of his 7-stage (stages numbered 0–6) developmental model. He stated in his original research that the final stage (stage 6) was rare. However, as there were few older people in his study, this is open to question. In research conducted since then, including MacKinlay (2001a, 2001b, 2006), numbers of older people have been identified according to his criteria, as meeting the description of stage 6. However, not all people do grow and change spiritually. Spirituality and/or religion is simply not important for some people, at any stage of their lives; others may have had engagement with religion and church as children, and fall away from this as adults; yet others come to faith or to a renewal of faith in later life. In this predominantly Anglo-Celtic and European group of participants, most are either Christian or have no religious affiliation.

As for other older people, those with dementia too may change in their engagement with spirituality, religion and religious practices. Fowler wrote of faith stages and that some would stay at stages 3 or 4. He called the final stage of faith development a 'universalizing' stage (Fowler 1981; Fowler, Nipkow and Schweitzer 1992). Where religion was seen in a more open and accepting manner, and doctrine and rules became less important, this may well have been the case for some in this study.

Most of the engagement with religious activities was either attendance at church services, or Bible studies. Some of the participants were very careful only to attend worship services of their own denomination, while others said that they 'go to every church service that is on', regardless of which denomination it is. The cohort of participants in this study have a history of stronger allegiance to particular Christian denominations than do Generations X or Y.

Amy, in the example below, attends as many services as she can; she also checked the facilitator, seeming to be critical of the facilitator's use of language in her question – did she 'enjoy' the service? Her response is clear: worship is not about enjoyment; it is more complex than that!

Facilitator: Yes, so do you take part in the church services here?

Amy: Oh yes, I go to all of them.

Facilitator: And do you find them, do you enjoy going?

Amy: Well, um, it's a hard question to answer because to enjoy is not what the faith is for.

Facilitator: Okay.

Amy: It's ah, well probably it is. (*laughs*)

Facilitator: (*laughs*) Well yeah okay, it, it's more complex than that.

Amy: (*pause*) Put it that way. But ah.

May is quite clear that she only likes to go to her own denomination services. A number of this generation of older people have remained loyal to 'their' church.

Interviewer: Yes, when you find meaning in life. What happens?

May: Yes, that's right, yes. Oh well really, I suppose my family and, it's tied up with them. And one thing we miss in here is not being able to go to church.

Interviewer: That's important is it?

May: Yes.

Interviewer: Yes, they do have church services here.

May: Well, not very often, and they are mostly Catholic. And we went once, and the person said we were quite welcome to stay but she could not give us Communion.

Interviewer: Well they should have Uniting Church services here, I think.

The following is an interesting position, where Margaret (MMSE 29) doesn't attend church but does go to and likes Bible studies.

Margaret: Oh yes, we all went to Sunday school when we were little.

Interviewer: Yes.

Margaret: And then church. Then I got away from church, but I like the Bible studies.

Interviewer: Yes.

Margaret: I'm not against, well I am against religion, I don't like religion just like it is.

In a number of Western societies, people will often acknowledge being spiritual, but not religious. Louise is another of the participants who no longer prays or attends church, but she seemed to be happy in the spiritual reminiscence group. The following is from her in-depth interview:

Interviewer: Now do you have really early memories in your life of say going to church or Sunday school or something like that?

Louise: Yes, I used to do that.

Interviewer: And was that good?

Louise: Yes it was. I don't do it now.

Interviewer: No? Do you go to any church services here?

Louise: Well I could I am sure, and might if I think, I have got a terrible pain of it, if I, kneel in fact, yes.

Interviewer: Yes. So you have got a pain in your knee?

Louise: Yes, yes, it is now. Talking it does.

Interviewer: So, do you take part, do you pray, or...

Louise: Beg your pardon?

Interviewer: Do you pray, or do you read any religious things at all?

Louise: No, I don't.

Faith had been part of the lives of some of these people for a long time, and in line with their current faith perspective, it was useful to consider the development of faith over the lifespan, where possible.

Interviewer: So your faith has been a part of your life from when? A long time?

Rodney: Yes, 1930, 1928 to 30, I can't think of the actual date, Billy Graham came to Birmingham, had a tent campaign, 10 acres, (*pause*) well I went to that, he was there for 10 days, I went to it every day, we did all sorts of work, everything.

Interviewer: Were you a Christian before?

Rodney: Yes, but I never proclaimed it. And while I was in there, he said does anybody have anything to say, so I jumped up, said I am a Christian, 'praise the Lord'. He said, got anything to say? And I said well, I have never come here before, but now, there was a thousand people in the tent, and I could honestly say the Lord is my Shepherd, saviour. Oh he was joyful.

Bronwyn spoke of her church attendance and also memories of church, and the importance she attaches to these now. In the excerpt below, Bronwyn also alludes to the support her faith has provided during times of need.

Bronwyn: Well I go to err the services as much as I possibly can.

Interviewer: So they're important to you?

Bronwyn: They are, yes. They are very much.

Interviewer: What would be your earliest memories of faith, church and so forth?

Bronwyn: Well, I still remember going back so many years ago, my mum and dad took us to church and Sunday school many times, and err. But I feel that somehow or other, I don't know how, why I feel that way, but He intervened. I was fortunate enough to be in the hospital when I had the heart attack, and the doctors were there and my daughter was there.

MAINTAINING CONNECTIONS WITH COMMUNITIES OF FAITH

Difficulties of actually maintaining links with communities of faith were raised. This is an important issue because numbers of these people were members of faith communities prior to admission to their facility. Although in many instances there is a chaplaincy team within the facility, there may also be a desire to keep contact with their long-standing community as well, if they live within a reasonable distance of their church.

Facilitator: Hetty, did you want to say anything about the church services, anything that's important to you at the moment?

Hetty: Well, more seem to be coming, don't they?

Daphne: Are you able to get anywhere these days, or can't you possible get anywhere?

Hetty: Oh well.

Don: If someone takes you.

Hetty: Yes.

Daphne: Oh, sorry.

Hetty: Well I, I can't get anywhere.

Daphne: No you can't do it on your own, no.

Hetty: No.

Don: Neither can I, as a matter of fact, unless someone helps me, because I can't see very good.

Daphne: That's why I am very pleased that I can just take my walker thing and go in the lift and I am there. I can manage. I would not be able to go out on the street, and go to a different church, but I am very happy with this.

Facilitator: Um, did you want to say something about the spiritual activities that you do, go to church, and things, and things that you do now, Hetty?

Hetty: No I, I didn't hear what you said, love.

Facilitator: Would you like to say something about, um, how important going to church is for you?

Hetty: Yes. I enjoy it. And there seems to be a lot more going to, to the church, that's not much, is it?

Facilitator: Is there one part that you like particularly?

Hetty: Yeah, yes, I like the, the…in the voice, I like the singing. I like the community singing too.

Facilitator: You do? You know a lot of songs, don't you?

HOLY COMMUNION

In one group session the participants were asked about taking Holy Communion, and their responses show the meaning and importance of it to them:

Facilitator: Communion, when you take Communion. What that means to you? How important is it?

Daphne: Holy Communion, the bread and the wine, yes.

Hetty: Well I, I feel different, having Communion.

Daphne: Mmm.

Hetty: I like it, I enjoy it.

Facilitator: And, Claire, can you, do you want to say anything about taking Communion?

Claire: No, dear.

Facilitator: That's okay.

Claire: Except that it has always meant something to me, deep down inside, it is a feeling you can't explain.

An idea of the image of God – a sense of what God is like

This was an important factor in meeting participants where they were in their spiritual journey. Critical questions related to what they thought God was like, if indeed they thought there was a God. The question to these people was not 'Do you believe in God?' but one step back, to ask what they thought God was like. This allows those who have no belief in God to say so clearly, while it also enables the interviewer or facilitator to explore with the individual their perception of God. Is it a helpful image that they hold? Is it an image that would support hope and spiritual growth, and even transcendence? These are all important questions when working pastorally with older people, whether they have dementia or not.

In this in-depth interview below, with Catherine, the interviewer explored the kind of image that Catherine had with her God, affirming the strength that this brought to her.

Interviewer: No. And, I wonder if you would like to tell me about the image you have of God, do you, what kind of a God is it, that you (*pause*)...

Catherine: We love God, and we worship when we can, and we don't like missing the church service if we can help it. It has got to be illness what made us miss it, and we carried that all throughout married life.

Interviewer: So that has been a real strength for you?

Catherine: Yes.

Mary, in the excerpt below, obviously felt free to express herself, but had difficulty in understanding the term used – 'image of God'. It is important to ensure that the words used are understood by participants. Even though the interviewer followed up with 'What do you think God's like?', it seems Mary was still trying to get a picture of God. This is an example of a person with dementia being stuck on the concrete term, in this case 'image', and missing the explanation.

Mary: Oh well I do believe in God, and I say my prayers. I go to church occasionally.

Interviewer: And what kind of an image do you have of God then? How do you think about God, what do you think God's like?

Mary: A nothing.

Interviewer: A nothing.

Mary: Absolutely nothing, I can't visualise anything.

Interviewer: Okay, you just have a sense of God.

Mary: Yes.

Enduring faith

For some, the religious habits of a lifetime still provide for present practice and comfort, as with Jennifer (in-depth interview only):

Interviewer: Um, well. Do you read the Bible? Do you (*pause*)...

Jennifer: I have got a prayer book, which I read occasionally, I will admit. I have got my prayer book, and I still say a couple of prayers every night before I go to sleep, and God bless yourself, so I believe there is something hereafter, I don't know what, we have all got to go somewhere, I don't know. I think religion is very personal thing. You either believe or you don't. I believe, that is the way I have been brought up.

Sylvia speaks of her family faith and affirmed her continuation of faith:

Interviewer: Ah hum, now I want to take a slightly different direction now and I wondering if you have ah any connections with faith at all, or do you have an image of God or...

Sylvia: Yes well actually, ah, just can't place when my faith sort of started like came into it but, ah I think there was always reasonable amount of faith because I, ah, my father was a Roman Catholic and I was brought up in the Catholic faith and, ah, my mother was, ah, I don't know if it was Anglican or what but she was ah, she wasn't a Roman Catholic, put it that way and, ah, if ah, Roman Catholic marries somebody that hasn't, is not a Roman Catholic, well it's a different attitude to in the home generally and, ah, I know that, ah, in later times I had quite a strong faith.

Interviewer: Yep, is that still with you?

Sylvia: Yes.

Interviewer: And is that important to you now?

Sylvia: Well, it's a hard thing to answer that because um, ah, I still have a faith, put it that way I still believe in, ah, in God, but ah, I don't think there was ever any real lack of faith, put it that way.

Interviewer: Yes, so it's just been a gradually growing thing through your life really.

Sylvia: I think it was, yeah.

Interviewer: Yes, and do you attend church services here? Do you go to Mass or...

Sylvia: Well they don't call it Mass because, ah, I think it is an Anglican faith they've got here now but, ah, I remember being really, ah, tied up in any one particular faith, I was just felt well, that God's God (*tails off*)...

Interviewer: Yes, so do you take part in the church services here?

Sylvia: Oh yes, I go to all of them.

Developing engagement with spiritual strategies and learning to connect with faith traditions

The range of activities of these study participants was narrow, largely, it seems, because it has not been the custom to encourage adults, and indeed older adults, to continue to grow in their faith. Of course there are a number of activities available, and pastoral care departments and activities staff can be proactive in developing resources in this area. As can be seen, even people with dementia may learn new things about their faith and about all aspects of their life and interests.

In the following discussion in one of the groups, it is also noted that it is important to offer possibilities that might be helpful to the resident in finding ways to support their spiritual needs, but at the same time it is also important not to proselytise. In this example, they are making suggestions to meet participant wishes regarding spiritual and religious activities that are available in the facility.

Facilitator: Are you sort of happy where you are in your spiritual life, Ben?

Ben: No, not really.

Facilitator: Aren't you? Hmm. How can we help, do you think?

Ben: Very difficult.

Facilitator: Hmm, yep. You would just probably like more contact with your, the church that you were brought up in. Well, we can talk to the minister and see if he can do something for you, can't we?

Ben: Oh yes.

Facilitator: Do you ever read the Bible yourself?

Ben: No.

Facilitator: Would you like to?

Ben: Well, I can't, I can't...

Facilitator: Concentrate on it.

Ben: Concentrate on, on it.

Facilitator: So you are better if someone else speaks to you about things, rather than you having to read it?

Ben: Yes.

Facilitator: Yes, hmmm. There is an Anglican Bible study on a Tuesday morning, you might enjoy that.

Ben: Oh, that is the, I wanted to.

Facilitator: June, June takes it, June the chaplain.

Anita: The chaplain.

Facilitator: Would you like to go along tomorrow, and just see what you think of it?

Ben: Oh, no.

Facilitator: You can be an observer.

Ben: Hmmmm.

Facilitator: Just sit quietly and observe, and see if it helps you at all, or is any use to you. We will have a talk about it tomorrow, see how you feel.

Amy: Excuse me again, is that the Anglican?

Facilitator: Yes, they have a Bible study on the Tuesday morning. You might like to go too.

Ben: And what did you say the name of the chaplain?

Facilitator: June.

Ben: No, I am lost.

Facilitator: Helen, our research assistant, is going to write it down for you. There you are.

Ben: June, yes.

Ritual, liturgy and art in the process of spiritual reminiscence

This chapter has provided an account of where these people with dementia have participated in worship, prayer and other forms of responses of ultimate meaning. Their experiences have been typical of people of their age group in a Western society: mainly the use of private prayer and attendance at church services. Spiritual reminiscence provides an opportunity to develop strategies for spiritual growth in later life. The process of examining meaning in life and then the way that each person responds to meaning invites a further step. That further step is to actually facilitate spiritual growth opportunities for older people. The churches have traditionally focused on the learning and spiritual growth of children, adolescents and young adults. It has often been assumed that adults do not need to continue to grow in their faith or to continue to grow and develop spiritually. Spiritual growth is possible until the end of life. Guidance and support to engage in new learning in later life is an important initiative to be developed. The process of spiritual reminiscence assists older people in finding their life-meaning; rituals, spiritual practices and liturgies help these people to continue a process already begun. In fact, rituals can become an adjunct to the spiritual reminiscence process, especially in a long-term group.

Rituals in the aged care facilities

Rituals are important for human beings; it is through ritual and the appropriate use of symbols that we respond to meaning. Kerrie Hide (2002) has written sensitively about the use of rituals and symbols for people with dementia. Goldsmith (2001) remarked on the importance of pattern that could even be affirmed through the senses; for example, familiar smells, such as the smell of bacon cooking on a Sunday morning in an aged care facility, that reminded elderly residents that today was the Lord's Day. Rituals can be whatever is meaningful to the participants; ritual should carry the meaning and affirm this within the participants. Niven (2008), for example, described the ritual that he worked jointly with an elderly woman to design, to assist her daughters to come to accept her approaching death and her gift to each of them of her rings. It was a simple ritual that empowered the woman in the process of saying goodbye to her daughters.

For members of the Greek Orthodox faith, the actual ritual with its rich sensory input may bring people with dementia into a special and sacred setting – bread takes on new meaning within the liturgy. The sounds and smells and sights within the service are deep with meaning. To an evangelical Christian, these rituals would seem strange, but to a member of an Orthodox

Christian church, rituals and symbols help them move into that sacred space of worship and awe. It is important that the type of worship is relevant to the people. It is stressed that worship is not about 'feeling good' but is a response to God that draws people into closeness of prayer and liturgy. The Holy Communion, or Mass, is an important part of this for many Christians, while for others, God's word through the reading of Scripture is the most important aspect.

Linking spiritual reminiscence with ritual

It is possible, once the group has been running for some time – for instance, after completion of the first cycle of six weeks of sessions – as they have grown in comfort with each other, that the group members may like to have ritual introduced. A good way to do this would be for marking special days, perhaps thanks for healing or improvement in health and well-being. Perhaps a group member has found new meaning in life through the process of spiritual reminiscence – celebrate it! The group can be involved in planning the celebration; might it involve thanks for life and hope? How can this be affirmed in ritual? The possibilities are open to the imagination of the group. The facilitator guides but does not overrule the group members; these things work best where the facilitator can allow the group to own the celebration. On the other hand, there will be times of sadness within the group when a member or someone close to a member has died. The group may want to honour the memory of that person with a small ritual prior to the start of the group. Birthdays and anniversaries are also special times to be affirmed through small rituals, as a preliminary to the spiritual reminiscence, and can in fact add to the reminiscence for that day.

Some groups may wish to begin the group session with prayer. It is important to keep in mind that these groups may consist of people who have a religious faith and others who have none. While all may feel comfortable in sharing the spiritual and religious beliefs and practices in the group, it is necessary to be respectful of differing beliefs and not to impose prayer on people who do not want it. Other specific prayer groups may be formed within the facility where prayer is the central focus of the group meeting.

Meditation

Moody (1995) has noted that growing older may be like a natural monastery, as older people tend to spend more time contemplating and reflecting on their lives; this is particularly so as they become more frail. A short and simple meditation session may be a good beginning to a session of spiritual reminiscence. A simple centring time is introduced, with the facilitator guiding the group in breathing deeply, becoming conscious of their breathing, and sitting in quietness for maybe just five minutes before the group starts. Meditation may be part of the pastoral process within the aged care facility, and it would form only a small component of the spiritual reminiscence session. It may be particularly helpful if the group members are restless when they arrive. Soft music may be played during their centring time. A balance is needed between introducing too many new things and providing a sense of security within the group. This is why it is probably better to not introduce too many new components to the sessions until the group has formed and people are relating well within the group.

Intentional linking of Scripture with reminiscence may be very valuable. Often older people have not studied Scripture in any depth, and the intentional linking of Scripture with the group member's life story can be growth producing. Depending on the participants' cognitive abilities, a process of using Scripture such as *lectio divina*, a way of prayerfully engaging with Scripture (Benner 2010), can be valuable. The use of art and music, or even holding the group session in an outdoor pleasant environment, may be conducive to quality reminiscence. The important thing is to maintain the focus of the group while adding interest and other ways of adding to the spiritual reminiscence process. This process is, of course, used appropriately, a powerful process for growth in its own right.

Summary

In this chapter we have examined the ways in which people with dementia in this study of spiritual reminiscence have been able to articulate their desires for worship, prayer and reading of Scripture, their memories of early religious activities, and their current belief and religious and spiritual activities. There are many examples of the religious and spiritual practices of the participants in the study. One point is made regarding the very traditional range of activities engaged in by most of the participants. It would seem that the assumption has been made that church services of worship are the main religious activity, and this is fine. However, there are additional ways with which to engage with the spiritual dimension and to grow spiritually in later life, and this would include people with dementia. Other ways of responding to meaning can be developed that will enhance their sense of well-being and to help them find meaning in the experience of dementia. The spiritual reminiscence programme itself is a valuable way of connecting with meaning. Other ways are in small group studies and the use of art, prayer and/or music to provide more opportunities for people to connect with meaning in their lives.

15

Designing a Programme for Finding Meaning

Throughout this book we have discussed the spiritual reminiscence groups and their outcomes. This chapter outlines how to establish these groups as part of the daily activities within an aged care facility. Much of what we suggest in this chapter has already been written about earlier in the book, and we will direct you to go back to read these sections in more detail. Also, there is a revised workbook being planned (to be published by Jessica Kingsley Publishers) which describes the process of spiritual reminiscence groups – you may like to go to that publication as well when it is published.

Who provides spiritual care to people with dementia?

In an aged care facility the question is often raised of 'Who provides spiritual care?' Theoretically, it could be seen to be the role of the pastoral carer. But is there any reason why spiritual care cannot be part of all care undertaken for those with dementia? Frequently we hear that because the person has declared no religion that there is no need to provide any type of spiritual care – and is this not the role of pastoral care anyway? So, how can spiritual care be incorporated into everyday care for older people with dementia? Having spiritual reminiscence groups is a way to undertake this. If we go back to chapter 1 we can review the value and role of narrative and spiritual reminiscence for those with dementia. Questions of what it is to be human are very important to these people, their relatives and those who care for them. If we view people with dementia as 'living dead' or less than human, as Behuniak (2011) suggests frequently happens, then what does this say about the carers for these people? Can carers feel proud of their chosen career if society so devalues the lives of those with dementia? These are very important questions, and they strike at the heart of how we treat elders in our society – Brooker (2004) describes this as dementia-ism – and it is just as pervasive as all the other –isms we are familiar with.

So, back to the original question – Who provides spiritual care? There is no reason why everyone working in aged care should not provide spiritual care. This ranges from the ethos of the facility to the day-to-day managing of personal care. Frequently we are caught up in the doing for older people with dementia and begin to forget the being of the person. We concentrate on what the person cannot do instead of what they can do – all these things add to the care of the spirit; if we planned all our care with the underlying philosophy of 'How can we help make these years meaningful for this person?' instead of 'How do we get through the chores of the day?' then we would begin to provide spiritual care. Kitwood (1997) has identified types of communication he calls malignant psychology – these include treachery, belittling, intimidation, infantilisation, banishment and stigmatisation. Many of these have been touched on already in this book – none of these can possibly enhance spiritual care.

A number of authors also identify that in order to meet spiritual needs there needs to be an overall atmosphere of acceptance. Peberby (1993; cited in Heath and Schofield 1999) suggests that the spirituality of the institution in which the individuals are cared for should be taken into account. The atmosphere and physical environment created by staff reveals much about attitudes to the total care of people. Father William Byron (1999; cited in Santora 1999) talks about how to reintroduce a sense of meaning into the workplace with what he calls the nine Pauline criteria – love, joy, peace, patience, kindness, generosity, faithfulness, gentleness and self-control. He believes that the workplace of today contains many of the opposites to these criteria – and this means the workplace does not have the physical environment that Peberby believes is essential for recognising the spiritual needs of older people in our care. We shall come back to this when we talk about some of the barriers to spiritual care.

Design of a programme

A programme of spiritual reminiscence requires a commitment from all members of staff in an aged care facility. As we have already said, nurturing the spirit takes place in an environment that helps to facilitate this process. From our own work, we have found that where the facility is committed then the spiritual reminiscence process is more successful.

In our present study we used two types of groups – one lasting for six weeks, the other for 24 weeks. In terms of relationship development the longer groups made more progress – participants developed supportive relationships with fellow participants. However, the length of the group may depend on the time availability of the facilitators. The length of each session tended to vary from 20 to 45 minutes. Session length was dependent on how discussion progressed – the groups with smaller numbers of participants tended to be shorter than those with larger numbers. From another perspective, we found that the longer groups tended to discuss in more depth each of the questions as time progressed – the basis of the sessions was a six-week programme that was repeated over the 24 weeks. If spiritual reminiscence was built into a programme of weekly activities (much like bingo) then there would be no 'end' to the programme – the cycle of six-weekly questions could continue with more exploration each time.

Group size also needed to be taken into consideration. In our groups we ranged from three to six participants depending on the level of communication difficulties and MMSE. In one group we had people from one ethnic background (see chapter 8) but in many others we had a mix of ethnicity. Perhaps more important than MMSE were communication difficulties due to poor hearing. However, facilitators who were aware of these issues managed the groups successfully.

The programme is designed to be presented over six weeks. Each week has a specific theme, and questions are related back to this theme. Although we give examples of questions to help with the discussion, there are many others that can be used – once the facilitator becomes more comfortable with the programme, more aspects of each topic can be explored. All the suggested weekly topics and discussion questions are in Appendix 1. Discussion seems to flow best when one question is introduced at a time and all participants are given an opportunity to contribute in turn, before introducing another question. In some cases involving people with greater communication difficulties, we noticed they would answer an earlier question later in the session. So it is important really to listen to the participants' responses and allow adequate time for a response. As we have seen from Killick and Allen's (2001) work, we may have to interpret responses and not just dismiss these.

Week 1 topic: Life-meaning

This week is important for settling in and getting to know each other in the group. Frequently, facilitators knew each of the participants prior to the group's beginning, but this topic often revealed more of the person with dementia than they had ever expected. When we interviewed people with dementia prior to starting the groups, they would say that they didn't have a story to tell, but once in the groups nearly every one of them did have contributions to make to the group.

The first week begins with a very significant question – 'What gives greatest meaning to your life now?' Experience shows us that many older people with dementia have little difficulty either understanding or answering this question. Some facilitators have tried asking questions like 'What gets you up every morning?' to elicit responses, but often these are taken quite literally and participants talk about breakfast! During this week we ask, participants about the joys and sadness they have experienced in their lives.

Week 2 topic: Relationships, isolation and connecting

The emphasis this week is on relationships. We have already discussed the importance of relationships and connecting in other chapters of this book – but it is here that participants are able to express their thoughts and feelings about these relationships. The session begins with a question like 'What have been the best things about relationships?' This is a good starting point for exploring relationships with the group. Think of a number of questions such as 'Who visits you?', 'Who do you miss?' and 'Who have you been especially close to?' We also explore loneliness and isolation this week – participants are beginning to feel comfortable together and in most groups are contributing well. We found that, for many of the participants, relationships were the most important things in their lives, even if past and present were sometimes confused; there was still a sense of 'knowing' and connecting that was deep and important. The relationship with their parents was in many cases particularly important, as was their concern for their partners, either living or dead.

Week 3 topic: Hopes, fears and worries

This week's session discussions about hopes, fears and worries can sometimes elicit a number of different responses from the participants. Sometimes this topic is difficult as the facilitator is concerned that people may become unhappy or distressed when talking about these issues. However, sometimes airing these fears made participants feel better – they came to a sense of peace they did not have before. We asked questions like 'What things do you worry about?' and 'Do you feel you can talk to anyone about things that trouble you?'

One of the comments showed that participants were relieved that others felt as they did and shared their experiences. Many of the participants talked about worries about the war in Iraq, financial issues or about their families. Some talked about the government or the lack of manners in younger people.

One group discussed the situation in Dili (East Timor) that had been in the news a few years before and identified ways they could provide some assistance. In an earlier study of cognitively intact older people, about 70 per cent of the participants named dementia as a potential fear for the future (MacKinlay 2001a). In contrast, the participants in this study had dementia, and it was generally not named as a fear. The importance of relationships was again stressed when participants spoke of whom they could go to if they had troubles.

Week 4 topic: Growing older and transcendence

One of the aspects of spiritual reminiscence is to get people to think about the changes they have experienced in growing older, whether through physical disabilities, psychosocial changes, role changes and/or losses. It is also helpful to reflect on how they are managing these changes and any difficulties they may be having, as well as the degree of transcendence they have achieved. Questions asked include 'What's it like growing older?', 'What are the hardest things in your life now?' and 'As you reach the end of your life, what do you hope for now?' We discuss the responses to these questions as part of chapter 5.

Week 5 topic: Spiritual and religious beliefs

This week is an exploration of spiritual and religious beliefs. It is interesting to talk about the meaning of God to these groups. They were brought up in an era when there was a greater participation in religious life, with 45 per cent of Australians attending church in the 1950s. The facilitator needs to feel comfortable with asking these types of questions. During this week questions about early memories of church are also asked. Some participants describe walking miles to church, or going to church when they were five years old with their parents. For those who do not have a religious background, questions about where they receive spiritual support or if they seek this support can be asked. Questions for this week include 'Do you have an image of God or some sense of a deity or otherness? and 'Do you find art or music expresses spirituality for you?'

Week 6 topic: Spiritual and religious practices

The discussion this week revolves around the spiritual and religious activities that participants are presently involved in. It is a good way to identify what people's needs are and whether these spiritual needs are being met. Many report prayer and reading the Bible as a part of their spiritual practices.

For those participants who expressed their spirituality through music, pets or the environment, we ask what they do now to meet these needs. Some of the questions for this week include: 'Do you take part in any religious/spiritual activities now? For example, attend church services, Bible or other religious readings or prayer, meditation or study groups?' and 'How can we help you to find meaning now?'

Training facilitators

The success of a spiritual reminiscence group rests greatly upon the facilitator. The role of facilitator in each facility is generally taken by the diversional therapist or activities officer. In some facilities it is the role of the pastoral carer. We have found in the research project that the facilitator needs to be committed to the concept of spiritual reminiscence. The role of facilitator in the facility seems to have no impact on this commitment – we have found that pastoral carers and diversional therapists make great facilitators or may have reservations about their ability to facilitate a group. However, like many tasks, the reminiscence programme works best when the facilitator is not just directed to take a group but feels comfortable helping people who may express loss, anger, loneliness, bewilderment or fear. We discuss the specific communication challenges of facilitation in chapter 12 – if you are on the beginning journey to a role in the spiritual reminiscence programme we suggest you re-read this chapter.

Once potential facilitators have been identified, there needs to be a structured facilitation training programme. This programme will equip them with the skills essential to managing a group. As part of this training all small group facilitators should first experience the process of life review and spiritual reminiscence. It is only by engaging in life review that facilitators will come to an appreciation of the value of the process. Facilitators need to feel comfortable with the whole discussion, and this life review helps the process. Other issues explored through training are specific communication strategies. These include many of the qualities essential for the helping professions and include: active listening; allowing participants enough time to respond; being empathetic; and recognising and responding to non-verbal behaviours.

Starting and establishing groups

Once the decision has been made to provide spiritual reminiscence groups at the facility and facilitators have been trained, then small groups can be established. Although in the present project we used spiritual reminiscence with those with dementia, it can also be used for older people who do not have dementia. We have found that, with groups of people who have dementia, it works best to assign group participants who have similar levels of cognitive ability to the same group; it may be useful to use the Mini Mental State Examination (MMSE) to assess cognitive levels. Sometimes, however, the MMSE does not seem to accurately reflect the ability of some people to contribute to the discussion, so a combination of MMSE and your knowledge of the resident gives the best outcome. With people who have communication difficulties, working with two or three people in the group may be sufficient. Finding a quiet place for the meeting helps participants to maintain concentration during the sessions.

A facilitator can work effectively with up to eight residents, but if any participants have hearing deficits, cognitive difficulties or diminished concentration span, the groups should be smaller. To overcome hearing difficulties the facilitator needs to pay particular attention to ensure that the person sits next to them and is included in all the discussions. One of the participants in our study was very hard of hearing and all group members ensured she was aware of the questions and able to contribute. We have found that, over the longer-term groups, the participants' abilities to communicate within the groups do increase, and it has been surprising to follow through the research findings for the six-month groups and see how the people have increasingly interacted with each other. This was often when their MMSE scores did not indicate that they would be capable of anything like the level of communication that did happen. Occasionally participants need to be excluded from the group work due to disruptive behaviours. In these cases, individual short sessions of spiritual reminiscence may be the most effective.

Challenges to the process

There can be a number of challenges to the success of the spiritual reminiscence programme. These can arise from institutional issues, lack of space, poor facilitation and stigma towards those with dementia. To ensure a successful spiritual reminiscence programme the institution needs to be committed to the concept. This means providing the facility and time for a diversional therapist to facilitate the group. The philosophy of care should include that those with dementia are not there to simply 'see out their days' but deserve the best care to ensure their final years are meaningful. Implementing this philosophy would ensure that there is adequate space for the sessions and adequate training for the facilitator.

Poor facilitation can hinder the development of the group. In chapter 12 we have referred to some instances where the facilitation did not enhance interaction in the group. The facilitator needs to consider all responses, help and support those participants with communication difficulties, use careful questioning techniques to help participants express their views, and steer clear of elderspeak and other patronising language. They need to use silence and allow enough time for participants to speak and be aware of interrupting or complicating questions. The stigma associated with dementia may prevent creative programmes being used to help enhance meaning for residents. If dementia care is built around reducing 'behaviours' then it is easy to overlook the core of the person and look for meaningful activities. When staff get caught in the daily chores of care and feel undervalued because of the societal approach to older people, especially those with dementia, then, again, meaningful activities are likely to be forgotten.

Spiritual reminiscence in international settings

Spiritual reminiscence is not just happening in Australia. During recent visits by Elizabeth to Singapore and Japan, spiritual reminiscence was able to be easily translated to these cultures – even through interpreters. In many Asian countries, where older people have greater respect and there has traditionally not been a history of institutional care, the care of people with dementia is relatively new. In the Asia Pacific region, only Australia, Japan and South Korea have public health policies directly targeting the issue of dementia (Parry and Weiyuan 2011). Spiritual reminiscence is a way of enhancing dementia care in these countries also.

Summary

Spiritual reminiscence is a relatively easy way to enhance meaning in life for older people with dementia. When we approach the care of people with the attitude of person-centred care based on respect and value, we can enhance the life of those with dementia and add another dimension to working with those with dementia. With strong institutional support and well-trained facilitators, it can be a very valuable addition to the care of those with dementia. Spiritual reminiscence translates well across cultures and can meet the needs of older person care in many countries.

16

Changing Attitudes and Empowering People with Dementia

In this chapter, we come to the end of the story of spiritual reminiscence as we have explored and developed it thus far. Where do we go from here? At a very important level, it seems to us that the work of Kitwood, back in the 1990s, was a crucial basis for the care of people who have dementia, and yet his work of person-centred care is still often only given lip service instead of being a real core component of care. To bring real change, nothing less than a cultural change is needed. What is needed now is attitude change in aged care facilities to empower older people with dementia. Cultural change is required throughout the aged care industry. Kitwood (1997) called for a 'cultural transformation' in dementia care. He described the new culture as one that:

> ...does not pathologize people who have dementia, viewing them as bearers of a ghastly disease. Nor does it reduce them to the simplistic categories of some ready-made structural scheme such as stage theory of mental decline. The new culture brings into focus the uniqueness of each person, respectful of what they have accomplished and compassionate to what they have endured. It reinstates the emotions as the well-spring of human life and enjoys the fact that we are embodied beings. It emphasises the fact that our existence is essentially social. (p.135)

We are convinced that spiritual reminiscence is a way of helping to bring about this cultural transformation in dementia care. To bring about this change there needs to be a focus, as Kitwood said so clearly, on the person rather than the dementia. Using spiritual reminiscence is a way of tapping into the core of the person in a way that does not usually happen in everyday interactions. We have discussed ethics and dementia in chapter 4, identifying the issues related to autonomy, justice, beneficence and non-maleficence, but also, most importantly, the attitudes and issues of the carer through the concepts of virtue ethics. To what extent do we 'protect' people with dementia versus empowering them by allowing them to make their own decisions? How can we change societal attitudes to consider those with dementia as embodied beings when so much of what is written about dementia refers to 'burden' or 'living dead'? In order to 'empower' a particular group it seems that someone else has to 'give up power' – how can we change care structures to enhance meaning in life and affirm the dignity and worth of the person with dementia?

In this chapter we challenge readers to participate in cultural change – we know that, in part, the cultural mores and stigma for dementia are accentuated because in our society we have definite and largely negative views of older people and people with dementia. Too often, we are worried about litigation, so we restrict the movement of people; we do not want to be embarrassed by displays of emotion, so we do not allow people to talk of sad things; and when people lose their memory we do not accord them the right of a story.

Challenging the myths and stigma of dementia

The myths of dementia are deep-seated within society. It is necessary to challenge unjust structures and the medical orientation of care that too easily labels people with dementia as being unable, focusing on what they cannot do, rather than supporting what is and can be possible. In this book we have challenged many of the myths of dementia. We have referred to books that have been written by people who have dementia. We have challenged the notions of 'burden' or 'living dead' and discussed the language that portrays dementia in such a negative way. Our participants in the spiritual reminiscence groups have challenged the notions that they cannot remember activities, that they are unable to respond to questions about meaning or that they are reluctant to speak of dementia or their own death. We have found that an MMSE score does not determine whether or not a person can communicate within a small group.

However, the myths seem to continue. Why is it that dementia seems to support continuing myths, even in the face of increasing evidence? One possible reason for this is fear. It is likely that fear underlies much of the myth, and myths, of course, support the fears, which are repeated and shared among those who know someone who has dementia. People are afraid of dementia because it is described as a 'living death'. Jolley and Benbow (2000; cited in Behuniak 2011) compared Alzheimer's disease with cancer, tuberculosis, AIDS and leprosy, since as a label it 'commands fear before sympathy, because it has been marketed largely through its most debilitating, demeaning and despairing features'. With images like these it is not surprising that people have a negative, fearful image of dementia.

As we have already discussed in chapter 2, the stigma of dementia makes it difficult for people diagnosed with dementia to talk about their condition. As soon as they 'confess' to dementia, their lives become defined by the disease, rather than by the person they are. The treatment of dementia, as a disease to be treated medically, has largely taken control from the person with dementia; the way back from this classification is hard and long. The social dimensions of dementia must also be recognised in the planning for and care of those who have dementia. When Christine Bryden (Boden), diagnosed with early-onset dementia, spoke publicly of her disease, some criticised her, saying that if she could speak, then she did not have dementia. As Christine remarked at the time, who would want to pretend that they had dementia? It is certainly not a fashionable disease.

One of the problems with myths is that people with dementia may well believe the myths of their disease and act accordingly. If you are afraid of the stigma of dementia, then you are less likely to seek help. If you believe that your life is no longer worthwhile or valuable, then despair and depression may set in – making all aspects of life more difficult. If you believe that people with dementia cannot manage daily activities on their own, then you are more likely to become dependent. If the people around you are afraid of letting you go out on your own, then you will stay at home. All of these myths can reduce quality of life and increase dependence but have no basis or evidence in fact.

'Behaviours' in dementia

If we are awake and conscious, we all exhibit behaviours all the time, yet people with dementia are often described as having behaviours – behaviours that are difficult. Much of the medical and psychosocial research in dementia has been about 'controlling or eliminating behaviours'. It is as if 'behaviours' have developed a life of their own! These 'behaviours' can easily become self-fulfilling prophecies, as the person with dementia struggles to make themselves understood by people who regard them as being incapable of understanding what is going on or expressing their wishes. There have been many reports of how the way that carers responded to the person completely changed the 'behaviours' – see work reported by Bird (2002), Kelly (2010) and Kitwood (1997). In each of these cases, scenarios illustrating 'problem behaviour' are completely different from staff member to staff member. Indeed, for some staff members, there was no 'problem'. It would seem that the problem behaviour was rooted in the care provided and the attitudes of staff towards those with dementia, not in the recipient of that care. Often the staff member's expectations of the behaviour will influence the way that the person actually behaves. Kitwood (1997) refers to malignant psychology to describe the negative approaches many carers (and sometimes society at large) have towards those with dementia. We have mentioned these in other chapters in this book. Kitwood's point was that what is understood by members of the medical profession as symptoms of the disease may in fact be the result of how people with dementia are treated, and how they are treated is the result of how the disease is socially constructed.

Empowerment
Empowering people with dementia
According to Goldsmith (1996), people with dementia are disempowered in two ways, first by the illness itself and second by other people's reactions to the illness. Empowering people with dementia is often about acknowledging what they can do, and giving them the benefit of the doubt, to allow risk-taking in circumstances that might have been restrictive or coercive. Martin and Younger (2000) describe a disempowering culture as one that is task-orientated, paternalistic and rigidly hierarchical, which would hinder or prevent a holistic approach to nursing care. Moves on the part of the individual carer to reduce the level of disempowerment would be almost impossible as the only way to change the culture would be to involve everyone in the workplace. Kitwood (1997) claims that in any organisation there is likely to be a close relationship between the way employees are treated by their seniors, and the way residents themselves are also treated.

Changing an organisation to encourage empowerment needs a complete rethink and reorganisation. The underlying concepts of spiritual reminiscence can form the basis of this rethink by encouraging cultural change that recognises the dignity and worth of all people in the organisation – regardless of whether they are a worker or a resident. Care of those with dementia would include recognising their identity and holding their story when they are unable to articulate this for themselves. Their story is vitally important, not just the facts of the story but also the meaning of the story for the individual.

Empowering families and carers
Empowering the person with dementia is vitally important, but likewise it is vitally important to empower the family and carers of those who have dementia. Families are affected by the same stigma that affects the person with

dementia. It is very difficult for families to come to terms with a diagnosis of dementia as they have heard so many stories of deterioration and 'living death'. Most of the studies undertaken into carer needs concentrate on the burdens of caring and the management of 'behaviours'. Kitwood (1990), when describing his malignant psychology, describes a vignette illustrating stigmatisation:

> Mrs D is known to be behaving strangely, and the ambulance has been seen coming to collect her to take her to the day hospital. The neighbours cease to show friendly concern and begin to look the other way. Relatives come to visit less frequently. The gossip goes around that Mrs D is 'going senile'. Children are warned to keep out of her way. (p.183)

Kitwood notes that the stigma of having a relative with dementia goes beyond that person and includes the whole family. He also believes that part of the stigma and depersonalisation that occurs for those with dementia is because we fear that one day we might be like that: 'to be with a confused elderly person is to be reminded, painfully, of one's own possible future' (p.185). This fear then leads to a psychological distance and a reluctance to get or remain close to them.

We have found that when we speak of meaning in life with those with dementia, the majority say that their family is the most important thing. It can sometimes be very upsetting for family members to feel that they are no longer remembered or are confused with others. Elizabeth mentions this when she used to visit her mother (see chapter 13); people would ask if her mother still recognised her, as if that would influence her visits – if she could not remember, then why travel all that distance? However, family members can help to maintain that identity for the person with dementia – who is better able to hold and articulate the story that is the person? It is up to family members and long-term friends to contribute to this.

Caring for a family member has many challenges and many rewards. In several studies it has been found that carers report positive benefits from caring. In one study of 85 urban caregivers, 81 per cent reported positive gains, including spiritual growth, personal growth and feelings of mastery, during the time they were caring for a relative with dementia. The same study noted that individuals who did not have a positive experience were more likely to be isolated (Sanders 2005 cited in Netto et al. 2009). Netto et al. (2009) found in their qualitative study of 12 participants that personal growth was the most common gain, including being more patient/understanding, becoming stronger/more resilient, having increased self-awareness and being more knowledgeable. Carers also developed deeper relationships with the person with dementia and 'higher-level gains', which included gains in spirituality, deepened relations with God, and a more enlightened perspective in life.

Finding meaning in the experience of dementia: The place of spiritual reminiscence work

We set out in this book to share the process of study we have engaged in over the last decade in working, especially with people who have dementia, on the trial and development of the process of spiritual reminiscence. We have distinguished between reminiscence and spiritual reminiscence by emphasising the meaning that is inherent in the process of spiritual reminiscence in contrast to reminiscence, which tends to focus more on remembering facts and events. Spiritual reminiscence goes to the core of what it means to be human; it explores meaning, in the context of hopes, fears, joys and the hard times, as well as spiritual and religious beliefs and practices, to bring a sense of fulfilment and joy to the final times of life.

How does spiritual reminiscence make a difference?

The importance of story for people who have dementia and for their families and carers has been an underlying principle of this book. If humans are biographical beings, and if our very identity is tied up in our life story, then to lose one's story is a devastating experience. This book has emphasised the possibilities of story and the ways in which people with dementia can and do retain their story through spiritual reminiscence. It has also shown that, when story can no longer be articulated, it can be carried by other people – by those with dementia, or by family members and carers.

Value for the people with dementia

We have written about the increasing vulnerability of people with dementia. We have outlined the difficulties of affirming people many would regard as being non-persons, or the 'living dead'. In this book we have shown that people with mild, moderate and advanced levels of dementia can be supported to retain identity. We have shown how connecting with story can be life-affirming.

SUPPORTING PERSONAL IDENTITY

Supporting the identity of the person through narrative or story is essential if we wish to really be serious in the provision of high-quality care. This is also essential if we really want to provide the opportunity for people with dementia to function to their optimum levels, to be able to flourish. We are convinced that the principles of spiritual reminiscence can support the continued identity and thus dignity of the person.

NEW FRIENDSHIPS

We saw that people in the long-term groups were able to develop new friendships through the membership and interactions that they developed with others in the groups. This is somewhat unusual in aged care facilities, where the concentration is usually on orientation of residents to the routines of the facility, the meal times, activities and other services. Little is intentionally done to create opportunities for the people with dementia, who have mostly lost all, or at least their most important, relationships, to form new friendships within the facility. Spiritual reminiscence provides a supportive environment in which this can occur.

FINDING MEANING IN THE FINAL YEARS

Using spiritual reminiscence is a means of helping people with dementia to find meaning in their experience of dementia. The questions of meaning that were discussed and explored with participants in the groups were well accepted by the group members. Numbers of them who could not usually remember what day it was would remember that 'this is the day for our group' and look forward to it with excitement. At the same time, many of these people found it hard to remember facts; it was only topics that had meaning that they were able to engage with and respond to.

Value for the carers

Carers of people with dementia who take part in spiritual reminiscence may find that participants are more at peace, and are more responsive and able to interact with them. The carers come to see another side of the person with dementia through their story, and this aids in the culture change that is required to give person-centred care. Carers may come to understand the reasons for so-called 'behaviours', and this will enable them to focus more on the person and less on the disease. This may involve changes to policy within the facilities to embrace the new culture for dementia care. For example, in one group that was conducted just prior to lunchtime, the group members would leave the session quite animated and go to the dining room, begin to engage others who were not in their group in conversation and find that there would be no response to their input. This put a quick end to lunchtime conversation at the meal tables, where residents had set places at which to eat. A programme of spiritual reminiscence and principles of spiritual reminiscence that went right across the facility would mean that not only those in a particular group, but all residents, would feel able to engage in conversation with others.

Value for the institution

Spiritual reminiscence affirms the dignity of the person, and this becomes an underlying principle of care throughout the organisation. If this occurs, then side-effects will include raised staff and resident morale and higher levels of satisfaction.

The pastoral carer role related to hope

The pastoral care provider may work with older people with dementia to assist them to find meaning in the experience of dementia. While the whole of the model of the spiritual tasks and process of ageing supports and guides the pastoral role, hope is so central to the well-being of the person that it gathers up the rest of the tasks into itself as this journey in hope continues. Hope itself may be fragile, and needs affirmation for continued well-being and to engage the possibility of flourishing. The pastoral carer works through the identified life meaning of the person to connect with this meaning. The role of the carer is to be present to the person and affirm their sources of hope. The pastoral carer identifies any issues that block hope and further spiritual growth, for example, grief, guilt and the need for reconciliation. The place of hope in dementia and dementia care has been tenuous, but spiritual reminiscence brings a positive contribution to facilitating hope in these people. Hope supports spiritual resilience and flourishing.

Spiritual care and spiritual reminiscence

While spiritual reminiscence is firmly within the role of the pastoral care provider, it is also an adjunct to the skills of all care providers in aged care and dementia care. These care providers can adapt their main practice modalities to incorporate spiritual care and the principles of spiritual reminiscence.

We believe that spiritual reminiscence provides a way forward to enrich the quality of care and way of life for older people with dementia. In this book we have shared the findings of over a decade of study and practice with people who have dementia and the strategies drawn from our work. We affirm the privilege of working with these participants of our studies and commend our work to your reflection and application.

APPENDIX 1

Group Topics for Spiritual Reminiscence

These questions are based on MacKinlay's spiritual tasks of ageing model (2001a, b) and were used in our studies between 2002 and 2005. A series of six themes of broad questions can be used to facilitate the process of spiritual reminiscence over six weekly group sessions. The questions below are the suggested outlines of questions for each weekly session.

Week 1: Life-meaning

- What gives greatest meaning to your life now? *And follow up with questions like:*
  - What is most important in your life?
  - What keeps you going?
  - Is life worth living?
  - If life is worth living, why is it worth living? If not, why not?
- Looking back over your life:
  - What do you remember with joy?
  - What do you remember with sadness?

Week 2: Relationships, isolation and connecting

- What are/have been the best things about the relationships in your life? *Use this as a starting point for exploring relationships with the group. Think of a number of questions, such as the following:* Who visits you? Who do you miss? Who have you been especially close to?
- Do you have many friends here? How many friends do you have?
- Do you ever feel lonely? When? *Follow up on things that might be associated with time of day, place, etc.*
- Do you like to be alone?

Week 3: Hopes, fears and worries

- What things do you worry about?
- Do you have any fears? What about?
- Do you feel you can talk to anyone about things that trouble you?
- What gives you hope now?

Week 4: Growing older and transcendence

- What's it like growing older? (For example, health problems.) Do you have memory problems? If so, how does that affect what you want to do?
- What are the hardest things in your life now?
- Do you like living here? What's it like living here? Was it hard to settle in? *And other questions of a similar kind.*
- As you reach the end of your life, what do you hope for now?
- What do you look forward to?

Week 5: Spiritual and religious beliefs

- Do you have an image of God or some sense of a deity or otherness? *Or, use other words that are meaningful to the group, such as:* What do you think God is like?
- If you hold an image of God, can you tell me about this image?
- Do you feel near to God?
- What are your earliest memories of church, mosque, temple or other worship? Did you used to go to Sunday school, church?
- Where do you go to get spiritual support?
- Who is the most important person to give you spiritual support?
- Do you find art or music expresses spirituality for you?
- Do you like plants and gardens, or animals?

Week 6: Spiritual and religious practices

- Do you take part in any religious/spiritual activities now? (For example, attend church services, Bible or other religious readings, prayer, meditation.)
- How important are these to you?
- How can we help you to find meaning now?

APPENDIX 2

Mini Mental State Examination scores for participants

Where two scores for each pseudonym are listed, the first listed is the first test.

Name	Score 1	Score 2	Name	Score 1	Score 2
Albert	29	27	Carol	27	
Alice	16	16	Catherine	16	
Amy	30		Christine	25	
Anita	13		Claire	22	
Annette	26		Daphne	30	
Ben	20		Dawn	18	
Beryl	17		Debby	16	
Beverley	23		Denise	25	
Bob	21		Dianne	9	
Bonnie	13	14	Don	29	
Brenda	NR		Dora	NR	
Brett	19	18	Doris	10	
Brian	19		Dorothy	19	14
Bronwyn	18		Edith	5	
Candy	30		Elvie	27	

Name	Score 1	Score 2	Name	Score 1	Score 2
Emily	18		Jane	30	
Emma	20		Janet	11	
Eunice	28		Janice	NR	
Eve	21		Jennifer	NR	
Evelyn	10		Jess	26	
George	NR		Jessica	9	
Gladys	22		Jill	3	
Glenda	26		Jim	NR	
Glenys	24		Joan	30	
Grace	25		John	25	
Graham	12		Josephine	15	
Gwen	15		Joyce	22	22
Gwenda	10		Judith	14	10
Hannah	12		Julia	22	
Heather	16	15	June	6	
Helen	11		Karen	12	7
Hetty	17		Keryn	20	
Heidi	12		Les	4	
Irene	6		Loraine	15	17
Iris	10		Loretta	NR	
Irwin	13		Lotty	29	
Ivy	4	6	Louise	4	
Jackie	0		Mabel	NR	

Name	Score 1	Score 2	Name	Score 1	Score 2
Madeline	23	26	Rosanne	21	
Margaret	29		Rose	19	
Marilyn	NR		Roslyn	NR	
Marjorie	NR		Ross	NR	
Martha	NR		Ruby	20	20
Mary	20		Sally	29	30
Matt	18		Sarah	14	14
Maureen	NR		Simone	24	29
Mavis	11	17	Sophia	NR	
Maude	12	14	Sophie	NR	
May	NR		Stella	8	
Melinda	NR		Sylvia	19	
Nancy	26	20	Tim	15	
Pamela	19	17	Tom	8	8
Peter	15	19	Una	19	4
Phillip	20		Vera	NR	
Regina	NR		Veronica	26	
Rodney	30		Violet	19	20
Roma	11		Zilla	12	
Rosaline	27				

Note *NR: Nil Recorded*

References

Abdalla, M. and Patel, I. (2010) 'An Islamic Perspective on Ageing and Spirituality.' In E. MacKinlay (ed.) *Ageing and Spirituality Across Faith and Cultures*. London: Jessica Kingsley Publishers.

Access Economics (2006) *Listen Hear! The Economic Impact and Cost of Hearing Loss in Australia.* Canberra: Access Economics.

Access Economics (2009) *Keeping Dementia Front of Mind: Incidence and Prevalence 2009–2050.* Executive Summary. Canberra: Access Economics.

Adamle, K. and Ludwick, R. (2005) 'Humor in hospice care: Who, where and how much?' *American Journal of Hospice and Palliative Care 22*, 4, 287–290.

Aged Care Standards and Accreditation Agency (2008) *Results and Processes Guide*. Parramatta, New South Wales. Available at www.accreditation.org.au, accessed on 30 November 2008

Allen, N., Burns, A., Newton, V., Hickson, F., *et al.* (2003) 'The effects of improving hearing in dementia.' *Age and Ageing 32*, 2, 189–193.

Alzheimer's Disease International (2008) *The Prevalence of Dementia Worldwide*. London: Alzheimer's Disease International.

Alzheimer's Disease Research (2011) *The Facts on Alzheimer's Disease*. Available at www.ahaf. org/alzheimers/about/understanding/facts.html, accessed on 21 June 2011.

Alzheimer's Society (2011) *Statistics*. Available at www.alzheimers.org.uk, accessed on 21 June 2011.

Australian Bureau of Statistics (ABS) (2007) *Census of Population and Housing Australia, 2006.* Cat. no. 2068.0. Census Tables. Canberra: ABS.

Australian Institute of Health and Welfare (2010) *Australia's Health 2010*. Canberra: Australian Institute of Health and Welfare.

Baker, D. (2000) 'The investigation of pastoral care interventions as a treatment for depression among continuing care retirement community residents.' *Journal of Religious Gerontology 12*, 1, 62–85.

Baker, R. and Dowling, Z. (1995) *INTERACT*. Research and Development Support Unit, Poole Hospital, Dorset.

Baker, R., Bell, S., Baker, E., Gibson, S. *et al.* (2001) 'A randomized controlled trial of the effects of multi-sensory stimulation (MSS) for people with dementia.' *British Journal of Clinical Psychology 40*, 1, 81–96.

Ballard, C., Gauthier, S., Corbett, A., Brayne, C., Aarsland, D. and Jones, E. (2011) 'Alzheimer's disease.' *The Lancet 377*, 9770, 1019–1031.

Bartlett, R. and O'Connor, D. (2007) 'From personhood to citizenship: Broadening the lens for dementia practice and research.' *Journal of Aging Studies 21*, 2, 107–118.

Bartlett, R. and O'Connor, D. (2010) *Broadening the Dementia Debate: Towards Social Citizenship.* Bristol: Policy Press.

Barzaghi, S. (2010) 'The Spiritual Needs of the Aged and Dying: A Buddhist Perspective.' In E. MacKinlay (ed.) *Ageing and Spirituality Across Faith and Cultures*. London: Jessica Kingsley Publishers.

Beauchamp, T. and Childress, J. (1979) *Principles of Biomedical Ethics.* Baltimore, MD: Johns Hopkins University Press.

Behuniak, S. (2011) 'The living dead? The construction of those living with Alzheimer's as zombies.' *Ageing and Society 31*, 1, 70–92.

Benner, D.G. (1998) *Care of Souls: Revisioning Christian Nurture and Counsel.* Grand Rapids, MI: Baker Books.

Benner, D.G. (2010) *Opening to God: Lectio Divina and Life as Prayer.* Downers Grove, IL: IVP Books.

Berk, R. (2010) 'The active ingredients in humor: Psychological benefits and risks for older adults.' *Educational Gerontology 27*, 3, 323–339.

Bird, M. (2002) 'Dementia and suffering in nursing homes.' *Journal of Religious Gerontology 13*, 3/4, 49–68.

Birren, J.E. and Cochran, K.N. (2001) *Telling the Stories of Life Through Guided Autobiography Groups.* Baltimore, MD: Johns Hopkins University Press.

Boden, C. (1998) *Who Will I Be When I Die?* Pymble, NSW: HarperCollins Religious.

Bowlby, J. (1973) *Attachment and Loss, Vol. 2: Separation.* New York, NY: Basic Books.

Brooker, D. (2004) 'What is person-centred care in dementia?' *Reviews in Clinical Gerontology 13*, 3, 215–222.

Brooker, D. (2005) 'Dementia care mapping: A review of the research literature.' *The Gerontologist 45*, 1, 11–17.

Brooker, D. (2008) 'Person-Centred Care.' In R. Jacoby, C. Oppenheimer and T. Dening (eds) *Oxford Textbook of Old Age Psychiatry.* Oxford: Oxford University Press.

Bryden, C. (2005) *Dancing with Dementia: My Story of Living Positively with Dementia.* London: Jessica Kingsley Publishers.

Bryden, C. and MacKinlay, E.B. (2002) 'Dementia – A spiritual journey towards the divine: A personal view of dementia.' *Journal of Religious Gerontology 13*, 3/4, 69–75.

Buckley, J. and Herth, K. (2004) 'Fostering hope in terminally ill patients.' *Nursing Standard 19*, 10, 33–41.

Butler, R., Orrell, M., Ukoumunne, O.C. and Bebbington, P. (2004) 'Life events and survival in dementia: A 5-year follow-up study.' *Australian and New Zealand Journal of Psychiatry 38*, 9, 702–705.

Chan, M.F., Chan, E.A., Mok, E. and Tse, F.Y.K. (2009) 'Effects of music on depression levels and physiological responses in community-based older adults.' *International Journal of Mental Health Nursing 18*, 4, 285–294.

Chenoweth, L., King, M., Brodarty, H., Stein-Parbury, J., *et al.* (2009) 'Caring for Aged Dementia Care Resident Study (CADRES) of person-centred care, dementia care mapping and usual care in dementia: A cluster randomised trial. *The Lancet Neurology 8*, 5, 317–325.

Chertkow, H., Massoud, F., Nasreddine, Z., Belleville, S. *et al.* (2008) 'Diagnosis and treatment of dementia: Mild cognitive impairment and cognitive impairment without dementia.' *Canadian Medical Association Journal 178*, 10, 1273–1285.

Chiu, J., Chen, T., Yip, P., Hua, M. and Tang, L. (2006) 'Behavioural and psychotic symptoms on different types of dementia.' *Journal of the Formosan Medical Association 105*, 7, 556–562.

Cohen, J. (2010) 'From Ageing to Sage-ing: Judaism and Ageing.' In E.B. MacKinlay (ed.) *Ageing and Spirituality Across Faiths and Cultures.* London: Jessica Kingsley Publishers.

Coleman, P.G. (1999) 'Creating a life story: The task of reconciliation.' *The Gerontologist 39*, 2, 133–139.

Corrigan, P.W., Watson, A.C., Byrne, P. and Davis, K.E. (2005) 'Mental illness stigma: Problem of public health or social justice?' *Social Work 50*, 4, 363–372.

Croot, K., Nickels, L., Laurence, F. and Manning, M. (2009) 'Impairment and activity/participation interventions in progressive language impairment: Clinical and theoretical issues.' *Aphasiology 23*, 2, 125–160.

Cumming, E. and Henry, W.H. (1961) *Growing Old: The Process of Disengagement.* New York, NY: Basic Books.

Damasio, A. (2010) *Self Comes to Mind: Constructing the Conscious Brain.* New York, NY: Pantheon Books.

Damianakis, T. and Marziali, E. (2011) 'Community-dwelling older adults' contextual experiencing of humour.' *Ageing and Society 31*, 1, 110–124.

De Leo, D., Hickey, P.A., Neulinger, K. and Cantor, C.H. (2001) *Ageing and Suicide.* Australian Institute for Suicide Research and Prevention. Canberra: Commonwealth of Australia.

de Vries, B. (2001) 'Grief: Intimacy's reflection.' *Generations 25*, 2, 75–80.

Dunn, K.S. and Horgas, A.L. (2000) 'The prevalence of prayer as a spiritual self-care modality in elders.' *Journal of Holistic Nursing 18*, 4, 337–351.

Edison, P., Rowe, C., Rinne, J., Ng, S. *et al.* (2008) 'Amyloid load in Parkinson's disease dementia and Lewy body dementia measured with [11C]PIB positron tomography.' *Journal of Neurological Psychiatry 79*, 12, 1331–1338.

Ekman, S., Norberg, A., Viitanen, M. and Winbald, B. (1991) 'Care of demented patient with severe communication problems.' *Scandinavian Journal of Caring Science 5*, 3, 163–170.

Emre, M., Aarsland, D., Brown, R., Burn, D. *et al.* (2007) 'Clinical diagnostic criteria for dementia associated with Parkinson's disease.' Movement Disorders 22, 12, 1689–1707.

Erikson, E. (1997) *The Life Cycle Completed: Extended Version.* New York, NY: W.W. Norton.

Erikson, E.H., Erikson, J.M. and Kivnick, H.Q. (1986) *Vital Involvement in Old Age.* New York, NY: W.W. Norton.

Farran, C., Salloway, J. and Clark, D. (1990) 'Measurement of hope in community-based older population.' *Western Journal of Nursing Research 12*, 1, 42–59.

Ferguson, J.K., Willemson, E.W. and Castañeto, M.V. (2010) 'Centering prayer as a healing response to everyday stress: A psychological and spiritual process.' *Pastoral Psychology 59*, 3, 305–329.

Ferri, C., Prince, M., Brayne, C., Brodaty, H. *et al.* (2005) 'Global prevalence of dementia: A Delphi consensus study.' *The Lancet 366*, 9503, 2112–2117.

Folstein, M.F., Folstein, S.E. and McHugh, P.R. (1975) '"Mini-mental state": A practical method for grading cognitive state of patients for the clinician.' *Journal of Psychiatric Research 12*, 189–196.

Fowler, J.W. (1981) *Stages of Faith: The Psychology of Human Development and the Quest for Meaning.* San Francisco, CA: Harper.

Fowler, J.W., Nipkow, K.E. and Schweitzer, F. (eds) (1992) *Stages of Faith and Religious Development: Implications for Church, Education and Society.* London: SCM Press.

Frankl, V.E. (1984) Man's Search for Meaning. New York, NY: Washington Square Press.

Gastmans, C. and De Lepeleire, J. (2010) 'Living to the bitter end? A personalist approach to euthanasia in persons with severe dementia.' *Bioethics 24*, 2, 78–86.

Geda, Y., Negash, S. and Petersen, R. (2009) 'Mild Cognitive Impairment.' In M. Weiner and A. Lipton (eds) *Textbook of Alzheimer's Disease and Other Dementias.* Arlington, VA: American Psychiatric Publishing.

George, D.R. (2010) 'The art of medicine: Overcoming the social death of dementia through language.' *The Lancet 376*, 9741, 586–587.

Gibson, F. (1994) *Reminiscence and Recall: A Guide to Good Practice.* London: Age Concern England.

Gibson, F. (2004) *The Past in the Present: Using Reminiscence in Health and Social Care.* Baltimore, MD: Health Professions Press.

Glaser, B.G. (1978) *Theoretical Sensitivity*. Mill Valley, CA: The Sociology Press.

Glaser, B.G. and Strauss, A.L. (1967) *The Discovery of Grounded Theory: Strategies for Qualitative Research*. Chicago, IL: Aldine Atherton.

Glaser, B.G. and Strauss, A.L. (1999) *The Discovery of Grounded Theory: Strategies for Qualitative Research*. Chicago: Aldine de Gruyter.

Goffman, E. (1961) *Asylums*. Harmondsworth: Penguin.

Goffman, E. (1963) *Stigma: Notes on the Management of Spoiled Identity*. New York, NY: Simon & Schuster.

Goldsmith, M. (1996) *Hearing the Voice of People with Dementia: Opportunities and Obstacles*. London: Jessica Kingsley Publishers.

Goldsmith, M. (2001) 'When Words Are No Longer Necessary: A Gift of Ritual.' In E. MacKinlay, J. Ellor and S. Pickard (eds) *Aging, Spirituality and Pastoral Care*. New York, NY: The Haworth Pastoral Press.

Green, J.B. (2008) *Body, Soul and Human Life*. Grand Rapids, MI: Baker Academic.

Hannemann, B.T. (2006) 'Creativity with dementia patients: Can creativity and art stimulate dementia patients positively?' *Gerontology 52*, 1, 59–65.

Harris, H. (2008) 'Growing while going: Spiritual formation at the end of life.' *Journal of Religion, Spirituality and Aging 20*, 3, 227–245.

Heath, H. and Schofield, I. (1999) *Health Ageing*. Trento, Italy: Mosby.

Hely, M., Reid, W., Adena, M., Halliday, G. and Morris, J. (2008) 'The Sydney Multicenter Study of Parkinson's Disease: The inevitability of dementia at 20 years.' *Movement Disorders 23*, 6, 837–844.

Herman, R. and Williams, K. (2009) 'Elderspeak's influence on resistiveness to care: Focus on behavioral events.' *American Journal of Alzheimer's Disease and Other Dementias 24*, 11, 417–422.

Herth, K. (1990) 'Fostering hope in terminally-ill people.' *Journal of Advanced Nursing 15, 11*, 1250–1259.

Herth, K. (1992) 'Abbreviated instrument to measure hope: Development and psychometric evaluation.' *Journal of Advanced Nursing 17*, 10, 1251–1259.

Herth, K. (1993) 'Hope in older adults in community and institutional settings.' *Issues in Mental Health Nursing 14*, 2, 139–156.

Herth, K. (2005) 'State of the Science of Hope in Nursing Practice: Hope, the Nurse and the Patient.' In J. Eliott (ed.) *Interdisciplinary Perspectives on Hope*. New York: Nova Science Publishers.

Hide, K. (2002) 'Symbol, ritual and dementia.' *Journal of Religious Gerontology 13*, 3/4, 77–90.

Highfield, M.F. (1992) 'Spiritual health of oncology patients: Nurse and patient perspectives.' *Cancer Nursing 15*, 1, 1–8.

Hogan, A., O'Loughlin, K., Miller, P. and Kendig, H. (2009) 'The health impact of a hearing disability on older people in Australia.' *Journal of Aging and Health 21*, 8, 1098–1111.

Holstein, M., Parks, J. and Waymack, M. (2011) *Ethics, Aging and Society: The Critical Turn*. New York, NY: Springer.

Hubbard, G., Cook, A., Tester, S. and Downs, M. (2002) 'Beyond words: Older people with dementia using and interpreting non-verbal behaviour.' *Journal of Ageing Studies 16*, 2, 115–167.

Hughes, J.C., Louw, S.J. and Sabat, S.R. (eds) (2006) *Dementia, Mind, Meaning and the Person*. Oxford: Oxford University Press.

Iadecola, C. (2010) 'The overlap between neurodegenerative and vascular factors in the pathogenesis of dementia.' *Acta Neuropathologica 120*, 3, 287–296.

Iliffe, S., Robinson, L., Brayne, C., Goodman, C. *et al.* (2009) 'Primary care and dementia: 1. Diagnosis, screening and disclosure.' *International Journal of Geriatric Psychiatry 24*, 9, 895–901.

Johnson, G.E. and Johnson, R.H. (2007) 'Implicit and explicit memory: Implications for the pastoral care of persons with dementia.' *Journal of Religion, Spirituality and Aging 19*, 3, 43–53.

Jones, W.P. (2001) 'In wait for my life: Aging and desert spirituality.' *Journal of Religious Gerontology 12*, 2, 99–108.

Kasahara, H., Tsumura, M., Ochiai, Y., Furukawa, H. *et al.* (2006) 'Consideration of the relationship between depression and dementia.' *Psychogeriatrics 6*, 3, 128–133.

Kelly, F. (2010) 'Recognising and supporting self in dementia: A new way to facilitate a person-centred approach to dementia care.' *Ageing and Society 30*, 1, 103–124.

Kenyon, G.M., Clark, P. and de Vries, B. (eds) (2001) *Narrative Gerontology: Theory, Research and Practice.* New York, NY: Springer.

Killick, J. and Allen, K. (2001) *Communication and the Care of Older People with Dementia.* Buckingham: Open University Press.

Kimble, M. (2004) 'Human despair and comic transcendence.' *Journal of Religious Gerontology 16*, 3, 1–11.

Kitwood, T. (1990) 'The dialectics of dementia: With particular reference to Alzheimer's disease.' *Ageing and Society 10*, 2, 177–196.

Kitwood, T. (1993) 'Person and process in dementia.' Editorial. *International Journal of Geriatric Psychiatry 8*, 7, 541–545.

Kitwood, T. (1997) *Dementia Reconsidered.* Buckingham: Open University Press.

Kitwood, T. and Bredin, K. (1992) 'Towards a theory of dementia care: Personhood and Well-being.' *Ageing and Society 12*, 3, 269–287.

Koenig, H.G., McCullough, M.E. and Larson, D.B. (2001) *Handbook of Religion and Health.* New York, NY: Oxford University Press.

Kovach, S. and Robinson, J. (1996) 'The room-mate relationship for the elderly nursing home resident.' *Journal of Social and Personal Relationships 13*, 4, 627–634.

Lesser, A.H. (2006) 'Dementia and Personal Identity.' In J.C. Hughes, S.J. Louw and S.R. Sabat (eds) *Dementia, Mind, Meaning and the Person.* Oxford: Oxford University Press.

Levy-Storms, L. (2008) 'Therapeutic communication training in long-term care institutions: Recommendations for future research.' *Patient Education and Counselling 73*, 1, 8–21.

Lichtenberg, P.A. (2009) 'Controversy and caring: An update on current issues in dementia.' *Generations 13*, 1, 5–10.

Lindberg, D.A. (2005) 'Integrative review of research related to meditation, spirituality and the elderly.' *Geriatric Nursing 26*, 6, 372–377.

Lipton, A. and Boxer, A. (2009) 'Frontotemporal Dementia.' In M. Weiner and A. Lipton (eds) *Textbook of Alzheimer's Disease and Other Dementias.* Arlington, VA: American Psychiatric Publishing.

MacKinlay, E. (1998) *The Spiritual Dimension of Ageing: Meaning in Life, Response to Meaning and Well Being in Ageing.* Unpublished doctoral thesis, La Trobe University.

MacKinlay, E. (2001a) *The Spiritual Dimension of Ageing.* London: Jessica Kingsley Publishers.

MacKinlay, E. (2001b) 'The spiritual dimension of caring: Applying a model for spiritual tasks of ageing.' *Journal of Religious Gerontology 12*, 3/4, 151–166.

MacKinlay, E. (2002) 'Mental Health and Spirituality in Later Life: Pastoral Approaches.' In E. MacKinlay (ed.) *Mental Health and Spirituality in Later Life.* New York, NY: Haworth Press.

MacKinlay, E. (2004) 'Humour: A way to transcendence in later life.' Journal of Religious Gerontology 16, 3/4, 43–58.

MacKinlay, E. (2006) Spiritual Growth and Care in the Fourth Age of Life. London: Jessica Kingsley Publishers.

MacKinlay, E. (2008) *Ageing, Spirituality and Disability: Addressing the Challenge of Disability in Later Life*. London: Jessica Kingsley Publishers.

MacKinlay, E. (2009) 'Using spiritual reminiscence with a small group of Latvian residents with dementia in a nursing home.' *Journal of Religion, Spirituality and Aging 21*, 4, 318–329.

MacKinlay, E. (ed.) (2010) *Ageing and Spirituality Across Faiths and Cultures*. London: Jessica Kingsley Publishers.

MacKinlay, E. (2011) 'Walking with a Person into Dementia: Creating Care Together.' In A. Jewell (ed.) *Spirituality and Personhood in Dementia*. London: Jessica Kingsley Publishers.

MacKinlay, E. and Trevitt, C. (2006) *Facilitating Spiritual Reminiscence for Older People with Dementia*. Barton, ACT: Centre for Ageing and Pastoral Studies.

MacPherson, S., Bird, M., Anderson, K., Davis, T. and Blair, A. (2009) 'An art gallery access programme for people with dementia: "You do it for the moment."' *Ageing and Mental Health 13*, 5, 744–752.

Mak, W. and Carpenter, B. (2007) 'Humour comprehension in older adults.' *Journal of the International Neuropsychological Society 13*, 4, 606–614.

Marston, D.C. (2001) 'Prayer as a meaningful activity in nursing homes.' *Clinical Gerontologist 23*, 1/2, 173–177.

Martin, G.W. and Younger, D. (2000) 'Anti oppressive practice: A route to the empowerment of people with dementia through communication and choice.' *Journal of Psychiatric and Mental Health Nursing 7*, 1, 59–67.

Martin, R. (2007) *The Psychology of Humour: An Integrative Approach*. Oxford: Elsevier Academic Press.

Martin, R. (2009) 'Humour.' In S. Lopez (ed.) *The Encyclopedia of Positive Psychology*. Oxford: Wiley-Blackwell.

Martin, R.A., Puhlik-Doris, P., Larsen, G., Gray, J. and Weir, K. (2003) Individual differences in uses of humor and their relation to psychological well-being: Development of the Humor Styles Questionnaire. *Journal of Research in Personality 37*, 1, 48–75.

Matsumoto, Y. (2009) 'Dealing with life changes: Humour in painful self-disclosures by elderly Japanese women.' *Ageing and Society 29*, 6, 929–952.

McCreaddie, M. and Wiggins, S. (2008) 'The purpose and function of humour in health, healthcare and nursing: A narrative review.' *Journal of Advanced Nursing 61*, 6, 584–595.

McFadden, S.H. (2004) 'The paradoxes of humor and the burdens of despair.' *Journal of Religious Gerontology 16*, 3/4, 13–28.

McFadden, S.H., Ingram, M. and Baldauf, C. (2000) 'Actions, feeling and values: Foundations of meaning and personhood in dementia.' *Journal of Religious Gerontology 11*, 3/4, 67–86.

McIntosh, M.A. (1998) *Mystical Theology: The Integrity of Spirituality and Theology*. Oxford: Blackwell.

Meacher, M. (1972) *Taken for a Ride: Special Residential Homes for Confused Old People – A Study of Separatism in Social Policy*. London: Longman.

Milne, A. (2010) 'The "D" word: Reflections on the relationship between stigma, discrimination and dementia.' *Journal of Mental Health 9*, 3, 227–233.

Minichiello, V., Aroni, R., Timewell, E. and Alexander, L. (1995) *In-Depth Interviewing: Principles, Techniques, Analysis*. Sydney, NSW: Longman.

Moltmann, J. (1967) *Theology of Hope*. Minneapolis, MN: Fortress Press.

Moltmann, J. (1991) *History and the Triune God*. St Ives: SCM Press.

Moniz-Cook, E., Stokes, G. and Agar, S. (2003) 'Difficult behaviour and dementia in nursing homes: Five cases of psychosocial intervention.' *Clinical Psychology and Psychotherapy 10*, 3, 197–208.

Moody, H.R. (1995) 'Mysticism.' In M.A. Kimble, S.H. McFadden, J.W. Ellor and J.J. Seeber (eds) *Aging, Spirituality and Religion: A Handbook*. Minneapolis, MN: Fortress Press.

Morgan, R.L. (1995) 'Guiding spiritual autobiography groups for Third and Fourth Agers.' *Journal of Religious Gerontology 9*, 2, 1–14.

Morgan, R.L. (2003) 'Small Group Approaches to Group Spiritual Autobiography Writing.' In M.A. Kimble and S.H. McFadden (eds) *Aging, Spirituality and Religion: A Handbook, Volume 2*. Minneapolis, MN: Fortress Press.

Morse, J.M. (ed.) (1992) *Qualitative Health Research*. Newbury Park, CA: Sage.

Morse, J.M. and Field, P.A. (1995) *Qualitative Research Methods for Health Professionals*. Thousand Oaks, CA: Sage.

Murphy, N. (1999) 'Physicalism without reductionism: Toward a scientifically, philosophically and theologically sound portrait of human nature.' Zygone: *Journal of Religion and Science 34*, 4, 551–571.

Murphy, N. (2005) 'Nature's God: Nancey Murphy of religion and science.' *The Christian Century 122*, 26, 20–26.

Murphy, N. (2006) *Bodies and Souls, or Spirited Bodies?* Cambridge: Cambridge University Press.

Museum Victoria (n.d.-a) *Journeys to Australia*. Available at http://museumvictoria.com.au/journeys/1940_60s.asp, accessed on 7 November 2007.

Museum Victoria (n.d.-b) *Origins: Immigrant communities in Victoria*. Available at http://museumvictoria.com.au/origins/history.aspx?id=36, accessed on 3 November 2007.

National End of Life Care Intelligence Network (2010) *Deaths from Alzheimer's Disease, Dementia and Senility in England*. Available at www.endoflifecare-intelligence.org.uk, accessed on 21 March 2012.

National Health and Medical Research Council (NHMRC) (2007) *Guidelines for Research*. Available at www.nhmrc.gov.au/guidelines/publications/e72, accessed on 1 January 2012.

Naue, U. and Kroll, T. (2008) 'The demented other: Identity and difference in dementia.' *Nursing Philosophy 10*, 1, 26–33.

Neary, D., Snowden, J. and Mann, D. (2005) 'Frontotemporal dementia.' *The Lancet Neurology 4*, 11, 771–780.

Netto, R., Goh, J. and Yap, P. (2009) 'Growing and gaining through caring for a loved one with dementia.' *Dementia 8*, 2, 245–262.

Neugarten, B.L. (1968) 'Adult Personality: Toward a Psychology of the Life Cycle.' In B.L. Neugarten (ed.) *Middle Age and Aging: A Reader in Social Psychology*. Chicago, IL: University of Chicago Press.

Nicholson, D.H.S. (1923) *The Mysticism of St Francis of Assisi*. London: Jonathan Cape.

Niven, A. (2008) 'Pastoral Rituals, Ageing and New Paths into Meaning.' In E. MacKinlay (ed.) *Ageing, Disability and Spirituality: Addressing the Challenge of Disability in Later Life*. London: Jessica Kingsley Publishers.

Norrick, N. (2009) 'A theory of humour in interaction.' *Journal of Literary Theory 3*, 2, 261–283.

OECD (Organisation for Economic Co-operation and Development) (2009) *Fact Book. Economic, Environmental and Social Statistics*. Paris: OECD.

Office for National Statistics (2005) *Focus on Older People*. Available at www.ons.gov.uk/ons/rel/mortality-ageing/focus-on-older-people/2005-edition/focus-on-older-people.pdf, accessed on 28 March 2012.

Oring, E. (2010) *Jokes and Their Relations*. Edison, NJ: Transaction.

Parry, J. and Weiyuan, C. (2011) 'Looming dementia epidemic in Asia.' *Bulletin of the World Health Organization 89*, 3, 166–167.

Pellegrino, E.D. and Thomasma, D.C. (1993) *The Virtues in Medical Practice*. New York, NY: Oxford University Press.

Petersen, R. (2004) 'Mild cognitive impairment as a diagnostic entity.' *Journal of Internal Medicine 256*, 3, 183–194.

Randall, W.L. and Kenyon, G.M. (2004) 'Time, story and wisdom: Emerging themes in narrative gerontology.' *Canadian Journal on Aging 23*, 4, 333–346.

Rayner, A. and Bilimoria, P. (2010) 'Dying: An Approach to Care from Hindu and Buddhist Perspectives.' In E. MacKinlay (ed.) *Ageing and Spirituality Across Faiths and Cultures*. London: Jessica Kingsley Publishers.

Royal Australian College of General Practitioners (2006) *Medical Care of Older Persons in Residential Aged Care Facilities*. Available at www.racgp.org.au/silverbookonline/2-1.asp, accessed on 23 May 2012.

Rusted, J., Sheppard, L. and Waller, D. (2006) 'A multi-centre randomized control group trial on the use of art therapy for older people with dementia.' *Group Analysis 39*, 4, 517–536.

Sabatier, P. (2003) *The Road to Assisi: The Essential Biography of St Francis* (J.M. Sweeny, ed). Brewster, MA: Paraclete Press.

Sacks, O. (1985) *The Man Who Mistook His Wife for a Hat*. London: Duckworth.

Santora, K. (1999) 'Spirituality in the workplace.' *American Association for Higher Education Bulletin 51*, 8, 3–6.

Saunders, J. (2002) Dementia: Pastoral Theology and Pastoral Care. Cambridge: Grove Books.

Seebus, I. and Peut, A. (2010) 'The Cultural Diversity of Older Australians.' In E. MacKinlay (ed) *Ageing and Spirituality Across Faiths and Cultures*. London: Jessica Kingsley Publishers.

Seeman, T.E., Dubin, L.F. and Seeman, M. (2003) 'Religiosity/spirituality and health: A critical review of the evidence for biological pathways.' *American Psychologist 58*, 1, 53–63.

Shiroky, J.S., Schipper, H.M., Berman, H. and Chertkow, H. (2007) 'Can you have dementia with an MMSE score of 30?' *American Journal of Alzheimer's Disease and Other Dementias 22*, 5, 406–414.

Sixsmith, A., Stilwell, J. and Copeland, J. (1993) '"Rementia": Challenging the limits of dementia care.' *International Journal of Geriatric Psychiatry 8*, 12, 993–1000.

Skultans, V. (2001) 'Theorizing Latvian lives: The quest for identity.' *Journal of the Royal Anthropological Institute 3*, 4, 761–780.

Smith, M. and Buckwalter, K. (2005) 'Behaviours associated with dementia.' *American Journal of Nursing 105*, 7, 40–52.

Snowden, D. (2002) *Aging with Grace: What the Nun Study Teaches Us About Leading Longer, Healthier, and More Meaningful Lives*. New York: Bantam Books.

Sorrell, J. and Sorrell, J. (2008) 'Music as a healing art for older adults.' *Journal of Psychosocial Nursing 46*, 3, 21–24.

Sternberg, R.J. (ed.) (1990) *Wisdom: Its Nature, Origins and Development*. New York, NY: Cambridge University Press.

Stokes, G. (2010) *And Still the Music Plays*. London: Hawker.

Strauss, A. (1987) *Qualitative Analysis for Social Scientists*. New York, NY: Cambridge University Press.

Strauss, A. and Corbin, J. (1990) *Basics of Qualitative Research: Grounded Theory Procedures and Techniques*. Newbury Park, CA: Sage.

Sullivan, K. and O'Conor, F. (2001) 'Should a diagnosis of Alzheimer's disease be disclosed?' *Aging and Mental Health 5*, 4, 340–348.

Sung, H., Chang, A. and Lee, W. (2010) 'A preferred music listening intervention to reduce anxiety in older adults with dementia in nursing homes.' *Journal of Clinical Nursing 19*, 7–8, 1056–1064.

Swinton, J. (2008) 'Remembering the Person: Theological Reflections on God, Personhood and Dementia.' In E. MacKinlay (ed.) *Ageing, Disability and Spirituality: Addressing the Challenge of Disability in Later Life*. London: Jessica Kingsley Publishers.

Tarawneh, R. and Galvin, J. (2009) 'Dementia with Lewy Bodies and Other Synucleinopathies.' In M. Weiner and A. Lipton (eds) *Textbook of Alzheimer's Disease and Other Dementias.* Arlington, VA: American Psychiatric Publishing.

Taulbee, L. and Folsom, J. (1966) 'Reality orientation for geriatric patients.' *Psychiatric Services 17*, 5, 133–135.

Tornstam, L. (1999/2000) 'Transcendence in later life.' *Generations 23*, 4, 10–14.

Tornstam, L. (2005) *Gerotranscendence: A Developmental Theory of Positive Aging.* New York, NY: Springer.

Trevitt, C. and MacKinlay, E. (2006) '"I am just an ordinary person": Spiritual reminiscence in older people with memory loss.' *Journal of Religion, Spirituality and Aging 18*, 2/3, 77–89.

US Census Bureau (2012) *Statistical Abstract of the United States, Table 77.* Available at www.census.gov/compendia/statab/2012/tables/12s0077.pdf, accessed on 21 February 2012.

Vis, J-A. and Boynton, H.M. (2008) 'Spirituality and transcendent meaning making: Possibilities for enhancing posttraumatic growth.' *Journal of Religion and Spirituality in Social Work 27*, 1/2, 69–86.

Viswanathan, A., Rocca, W. and Tzourio, C. (2009) 'Vascular risk factors and dementia: How to move forward.' *Neurology 72*, 4, 368–374.

Wall, M. and Duffy, A. (2010) 'The effects of music therapy for older people with dementia.' *British Journal of Nursing 19*, 2, 108–113.

Weaver, G. (2004) 'Embodied Spirituality: Experiences of Identity and Spiritual Suffering Among Persons with Alzheimer's Dementia.' In M. Jeeves (ed.) *From Cells to Souls and Beyond.* Grand Rapids, MI: Eerdmans.

Webster, J.D. and Haight, B.K. (eds) (2002) *Critical Advances in Reminiscence Work: From Theory to Application.* New York, NY: Springer.

Werner, P. and Heinik, J. (2008) 'Stigma by association and Alzheimer's disease.' *Aging and Mental Health 12*, 1, 92–99.

Werrell, R.S. (2006) *The Theology of William Tyndale.* Cambridge: James Clarke & Co.

Williams, K., Herman, R., Gajewski, B. and Wilson, K. (2009) 'Elderspeak communication: Impact on dementia care.' *American Journal of Alzheimer's Disease and Other Dementias 24*, 11, 11–20.

Wolverson (Radbourne), E.L., Clarke, C. and Moniz-Cook, E. (2010) 'Remaining hopeful in early-stage dementia: A qualitative study.' *Aging and Mental Health 4*, 14, 450–460.

Woods, R.T. (1989) Alzheimer's Disease: Coping with a Living Death. London: Souvenir Press.

Woods, R.T. (1999) 'The person in dementia care.' *Generations 23*, 3, 35–39.

Yale, R. (1995) *Developing Support Groups for Individuals with Early-Stage Alzheimer's Disease: Planning, Implementation and Evaluation.* Baltimore, MD: Health Professions Press.

Subject Index

Author Index

Made in the USA
Middletown, DE
31 July 2016